Accelerated Stroke Recovery

by Helen Randall

Recover from Your Stroke Rapidly and Easily

The information in this book will help accelerate your recovery from a stroke and help avoid the doldrums and frustration many people experience during post-stroke rehab. This book will increase your motivation. **It is organized so that you can head directly to the information you need.**

An All-Bullet-Points Book!
Consume Content Quickly!
Easy!   Fast!   Efficient!

You are undoubtedly familiar with the experience of reading a lengthy book only to find that it actually contained a relatively small amount of highly useful information that was buried among a copious amount of filler material. You ended up reading 200 pages and highlighted maybe fifteen percent—the valuable relevant information you were searching for. Was the author hoping to impress you with substantial volume? The time spent reading extraneous information was essentially wasted.

In this bullet-format book I have focused only on the most useful and dynamic information. **I have omitted the filler, organized the content and focused on the information you will need to gain the most help in the shortest reading time.**

Contents

What Happened to Me?

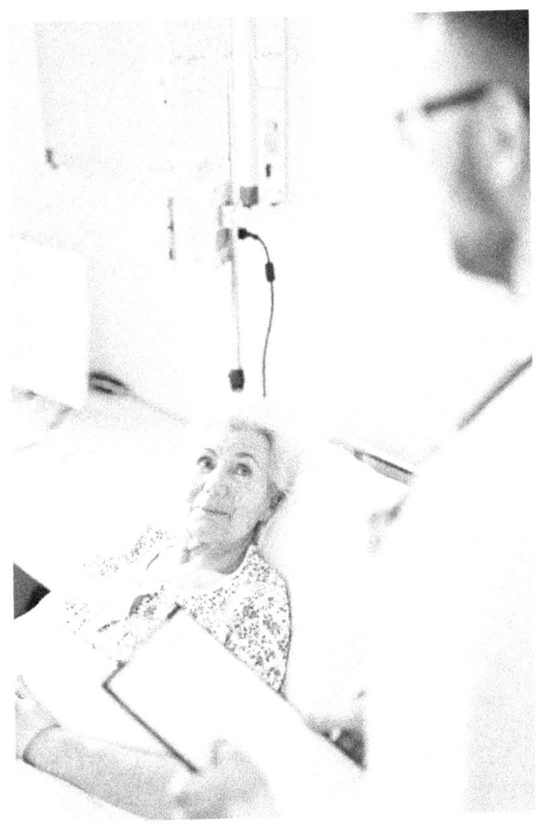

- If you're reading this, you probably had a stroke.

- After a stroke you are likely to experience a variety of symptoms that can include drooping on one side of the face, weakness or numbness in your arm on the affected side and an inability to lift that arm, slurred speech or an inability to talk, weakness or even paralysis of the body along one side.

- Some stroke patients experience impaired vision, dizziness, confusion or difficulty understanding other people, loss of balance and coordination, and difficulty swallowing.

- Your stroke could have happened in one of two ways: 87% of strokes are ischemic stroke caused by the blockage of a blood vessel in your brain by a clot or plaque, resulting in damage to a part of your brain that was shut off from oxygen.[47, 48]

- The remaining 13% are hemorrhagic strokes are caused when an artery wall in the brain ruptures, usually as a result of high blood pressure. This rupture causes damage to the surrounding area.[1, 47, 48.]

- Was your stroke a bleed or a clog? The type of stroke you had, and the side of the brain in which it occurred, can affect your symptoms and recovery time.

- Every stroke is unique, depending on which part of the brain was damaged. A stroke in one side of the brain will affect the other side of the body.

- Because each side of the brain controls different neurological faculties, it is possible to predict symptoms based on the location of the stroke.

- If your stroke occurred in the brain's right side, the left side of your body will probably be affected by weakness or even paralysis. If the stroke occurred in the brain's left side, the right side will become weak or paralyzed.

- Right brain stroke symptoms include poor balance, vision problems, difficulty moving, poor eye-hand coordination, extreme exhaustion, and too much or too little muscle tone (spasticity or flaccidity) in seemingly random areas.

- Psychological effects of right brain strokes include impulsive behavior, becoming impatient easily, and memory loss. [1, 25]

- If your stroke occurred in the left side of your brain, the right side of your body will likely be affected by weakness or paralysis. You may also have speech problems, slow thinking, cautious behavior, and impaired memory.[1, 25.]

- A combination of time, treatment, and active participation on your part will cause you to improve significantly. [1]

- Researchers now liken having a stroke to suddenly unplugging a computer. Your brain has been functioning non-stop ever since you became conscious.

- When the stroke happened, connections between nerves and muscles were lost, and now they need to be reconnected and reignited.

- In the year after a stroke, about 10 percent of patients die, have another stroke, or heart attack, or are admitted to a long-

term care facility. You can avoid another stroke or heart attack
with positive lifestyle changes

- You survived your stroke, and now medical science knows that
the brain can heal after a stroke.

- Twenty years ago, we didn't have the excellent after-stroke
rehab we do today. So put things in perspective, get on with
your life and focus on gratitude rather than being a victim.

Get Moving! Right Away!

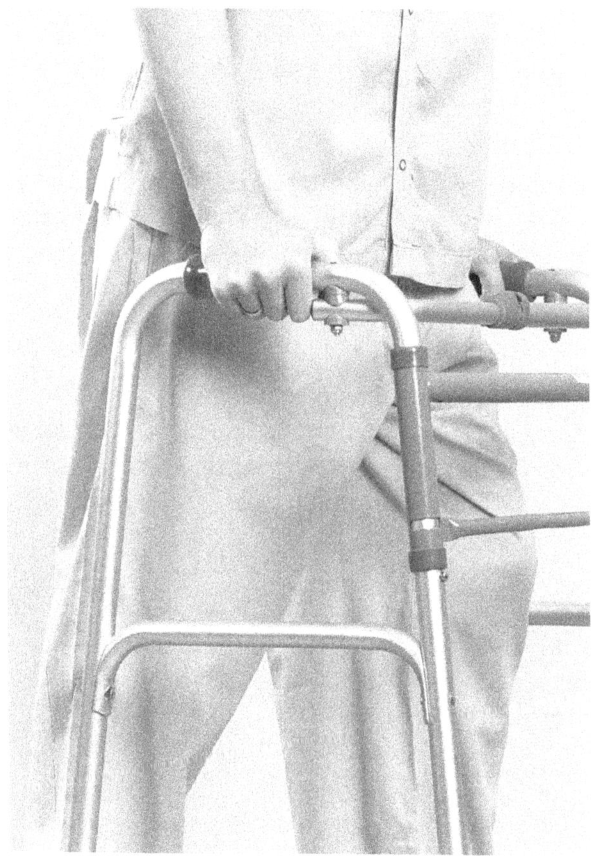

- The sooner you start moving the sooner you will regain lost abilities and skills.

- It's common for stroke rehabilitation to start as soon as 24 to 48 hours after your stroke. It's essential to get moving in order to reactivate the links between the brain and peripheral nerves and muscles.

- After your stroke your doctors' immediate priorities are to stabilize your medical condition, control life-threatening conditions, prevent another stroke, and limit any stroke-related complications.

- Obviously you will need to have some rest and let your body recover after your stroke, but if you are very sedentary and don't get out of bed, your muscles can atrophy and contract, and you run the risk of contracture or immobility.

- Repetitive movement promotes neuroplasticity which is the brain's ability to reconnect the neuron (nerve) links that were damaged by the stroke with your muscles. Effective physical therapy is the way to regain mastery of your body.

- The part of your brain affected by the stroke will probably not repair itself, but with repetitive movement, the surrounding neurons will rise to the occasion, creating new nerve pathways to restore neuroplasticity.

- Move. Then move some more. You need to teach those leg, arm and shoulder muscles to move again, and that is going to be done by moving them—in ever increasing ranges of motion.

- Just because you find it harder to get around, doesn't mean you can't get stronger and improve coordination with an appropriate exercise program provided for you through physical and occupational therapy.

- Stroke patients who follow through on their rehab exercises are able to renew the brain-muscle links and regain a significant percentage, if not all, of the mobility they had before their stroke.

- One commonly recognized syndrome in stroke recovery, is a tendency to just do nothing and wait for the condition to get better by itself. This is an easy path to follow, but it's not going to help.

- The only way to get your muscles working is to move them and re-establish nerve-muscle connections.

- Keep in mind that exercise will also help you stay mentally sharp.

- When you consider that many stroke patients simply leave the hospital, buy an electric wheelchair, figuring that's an easy way to become mobile and don't do any physical therapy at all, it is no wonder that leveling off occurs for many of these patients.

- Some patients purchase expensive electronic aids, but they generally don't work better than repetitive exercise and the use of resistance bands, weights and other aids to assist recovery.

- In most cases neuroplasticity and strength can be fully restored with repetitive exercise.

- Repetition of movement is the dynamo that restores control.

- Your leg will heal first because you'll automatically do more weight-bearing exercise. Arm and shoulder control will follow but lots of repetitive movement is necessary for a full recovery.

- As soon as possible, even while you're in the hospital, start doing a little weight-bearing exercise with your weak arm. Try to use that arm to help lift yourself up to a sitting position.

- Physical therapists have found that healing occurs faster in those patients whose weak arm is on the same side as the entry to the room. You will heal faster if you push yourself up with that weak arm.

- Physical therapy focused on the weak arm can make a big difference. Keep your arm moving. Stretch your fingers wide. Make a fist often. Move your wrist from side to side and up and down.

- You need to loosen up rigid muscles that are impeding mobility.

- Your body needs to discover that being on vacation isn't going to cut it. Remember you are the boss.

- Practice straightening your weak arm at the elbow. Your brain is trying to protect you since you have just experienced a major trauma. So your arm will tend to curl back into your body in a defensive position.

- You can override arm curl by making it a point to straighten your arm when you are sitting, walking or lying in bed.

- Make an effort to extend your range of wrist movement. Hold your hand out palm up in front of you (supination) and turn it over (pronation). Also lower and raise your hand at the wrist. Get your shoulder moving again by raising your arm.

- The exercises that will help you the most are pretty easy. Doing weight-bearing exercises with your weak arm will help you get out of a car, and marching while seated (lifting your knees high) will strengthen your thighs and help you get up from a sitting position.

- You may be advised to use constraint-induced therapy where your unaffected limb is restrained while you practice moving the affected limb to help improve its function. This type of therapy is sometimes called "forced-use therapy."

- Range-of-motion therapy focuses on exercises and treatments that can loosen muscle tension (spasticity) and help you increase the range of motion in areas that are stiff. Apply heat and ice on stiff muscles.

- Increase the range of motion in your hand by straightening your fingers and pulling your fingers apart sideways. Clench your fist and rotate your wrist.

- Increase the range of motion of your shoulder by doing shoulder circles. A mini hand-bicycle can be helpful.

- Motor-skill exercises will help improve your muscle strength and coordination and enhance neuroplasticity and motor development. Focus on your weak areas.

- You'll have to set aside a designated time. Otherwise distraction will intervene.

- Consistency trumps strenuous workouts done spasmodically. Continuous light exercise is much more beneficial than spurts of high energy activity.

- Plan your day around episodes of therapeutic movement. You eat on a schedule, so exercise on a schedule. And remember, repetitive movement is just as important for your recovery as your meals are.

- Do your rehab exercises before or after you eat, or before bed, so that a rhythm starts forming in your daily schedule.

- Prioritize your daily walks. A couple of short walks per day are more beneficial than one long exhausting walk.

- If you over-exert yourself, you'll find that you'll probably lose some motor control, your weakened foot will tend to drag, and you may experience stiffness and lack of coordination.

- Schedule a walk when you wake up in the morning and get it done before distraction sidetracks you.

- Mobility training will help you learn to use a mobility aid such as a wheelchair, a walker, a quad-cane, or an ankle brace. The ankle brace can stabilize and strengthen your ankle to help support your body's weight while you relearn to walk.

- It may seem to be slow going, but you'll recover a lot of movement in the first few weeks.

- Make sure to cover some distance each day with your mobility aid. You might want to use trekking poles rather than a cane to aid in stability and give your arms and legs a workout.

- Realize that even if you are limited to a wheelchair, you can do some exploring. But try to avoid inclines. Once you graduate to a walker or a rollator, a daily outing will do wonders. A walk in the park can be enjoyable and help you get stronger.

- After you walk, your muscles will be less stiff, so that's a great time to do stretches with your legs. Stretching will help condition your muscles and accelerate your progress.

- While lying down, lift your weak leg. Bend your knee and slowly, in a controlled manner, move your leg towards and away from your torso. Also move your knee from side to side.

- You will make good progress with just 5 minutes of leg exercises per day.

- The process of stroke recovery is very similar to learning an instrument, where it is necessary to practice repetitive patterns of very fine motor skills.

- When learning a new skill, it is common to meet with your teacher approximately once a week and be given instructions to practice each day until the next lesson. The same applies to stroke recovery.

- Your speed of recovery will be highly affected by the amount of dedication and practice of physical therapy techniques. The more you do, the faster you'll recover.

- You may be surprised at how quickly the tasks will become easier as you practice repetitions of the same movements, reestablish nerve-muscle connections and restore movement in muscles that have become atrophied from inactivity.

- It may seem like your progress should be faster, but to others you are probably doing well. So be patient. A practice session daily will improve your mobility, your range of movement, and your confidence.

- Try to avoid comparing yourself with other stroke survivors. There are so many variables. The brain is extremely complex and depending on which area of the brain was injured, the affected part of the body will vary.

- Keep in mind, some patients are older, some younger, some fitter, some way out of shape. Every stroke survivor has a unique history and will progress at his or her own rate.

- Make it easy to exercise by wearing clothes that are easy to put on and take off. Tops should open at the front. Zippers and Velcro are easier to open and close than buttons are.

- Shorts and pants should have elastic at the waist so they can be pulled up easily.

- When putting on pants, insert your affected foot first and leave your strong foot free for balance. When taking off your pants, free your good foot first in case you lose your balance.

- Wear Velcro sneakers or put elastic laces in your sneakers so you don't have to tie any laces. Always wear sox to avoid blisters, especially if you are diabetic. Liner sox are easier to put on than long sox.

- Trust your physical and occupational therapists. They've studied physiology for years. They know which muscles need to be worked in order for you to regain strength and coordination.

- Even though your therapists' guidance may seem repetitive, over-protective and limiting, they have an obligation to protect you from a fall which could seriously injure you, or set you back.

- Use props. While sitting, push your weight down on your cane with your weak hand. Stretch your shoulder by rotating the anchored cane in a circular motion.

- Tie a resistance band for strengthening your weak arm to an easily accessible door handle.

- Always stop as soon as it starts to hurt.

- A one or two pound weight is useful for rotating your affected wrist. Not too heavy, but heavy enough for the muscles to detect some resistance.

- See if you can do full rotations from palm up to palm down and while holding a weight, raise your clenched wrist back towards your elbow to increase range of motion.

- If your weak hand and wrist are swollen with edema caused by inflammation, this will limit movement. The swelling can often be reduced by applying a cold pack.

- To increase range of movement in your shoulder, attach a specialized pulley for stroke rehab to the top of a door and leave in place a stool or chair handy to sit while using it.

- You can also hold on to your cane with both hands, about 2 feet apart, and lift your weak arm up over your head with your strong arm to the point at which you begin to detect pain. 15 reps a day can help.

- Increased range of motion will probably be noticeable after just a few days of practice.

- Do 20 repetitions with your pulley or cane before bed and when you get up in the morning.

- After you've done your arm-raising exercises, lie down and again lift both arms up and back using your cane or a dowel. It will be easier after you've loosened your shoulder muscles with the pulley.

- It's good to anchor your elbows on the bed so that they touch your waist and using the cane, push your weak arm away from your body with your strong arm. This will really help with range of motion.

- When you can extend out your weak arm from the shoulder, bent at the elbow and flap it like a chicken wing, you're making great progress. When you can extend your arm in front, even better.

- Sit in front of a mirror when you're lifting your arms or shoulders, to make sure you're not dropping the shoulder on your weakened side. You can also use your strong arm to lift your weak arm to the front. But always stop immediately if it starts to hurt.

- The exercises demonstrated and taught by physical therapists are scientifically designed to efficiently re-establish the links from brain to muscle that are necessary for full rehabilitation.

- Health practitioners have noted that after a few months, some stroke patients tend to level off in terms of regaining motor function because they stop practicing their physical therapy exercises when their sessions end.

- Patients who continue to do their physical therapy exercises make good progress.

- When your physical and occupational therapy comes to an end, it is extremely important that you keep up with the rehab exercises. Set a specific time aside each day to practice the exercises you have learned.

- You may find that some of the physical therapy exercises you stopped doing weeks ago are actually more valuable than you thought they were, especially if you notice symptoms returning. If your foot starts to drop again, for example, do the exercises that help you raise your toe.

- Remember, you have to keep up your training. Even the best golfers in the world practice daily. If you don't keep up with your exercises you may find yourself becoming weaker.

- If you do find yourself spending hours lying down each day, get up and walk for a minute or two every 45 minutes. This will help your flexibility and strength.

- Stay active on a daily basis. Go out. Use your walker or rollator to walk around the mall, a farmers market, the park, or a superstore.

- You'll find that the more stimulating your visual environment is, the easier it will be for you to stay on your feet longer, because your interest will motivate you to keep going.

- Once you become more mobile, you'll be able to appreciate a little more of what the world has to offer. Visualize the life you really want and then work relentlessly towards making it a reality.

- There is so much out there in this beautiful world to see and discover. But it depends on how much consistency you are willing to apply in order to get your functionality back. So go for it. You have so much to gain and virtually nothing to lose.

Accelerating the Healing Process

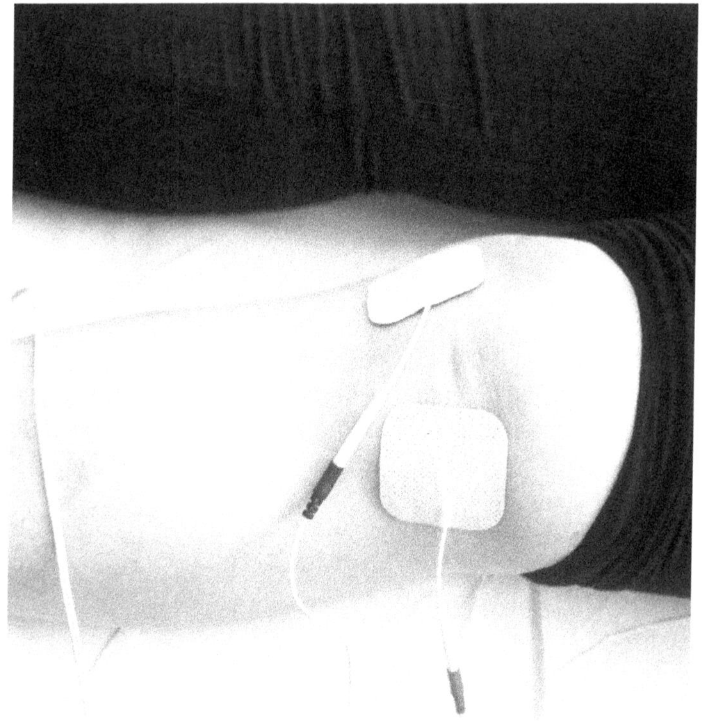

- With strategic techniques you can accelerate the speed of rehabilitation and get back to where you were pre-stroke.

- There are now some methods available that can help speed up the time it takes to get muscles working again.

- Some stroke recovery centers are using electric muscle stimulation (EMS), also known as neuromuscular electrical stimulation to strengthen muscles and speed up recovery.

- No matter how quickly you want to return to your pre-stroke condition, it's important to be aware that healing will take time, just as an injury takes time to heal.

- Relax. Be patient. it's imperative to accept the fact that muscles have to strengthen. Nerve connections need time to grow.

- Depending on how fit you were before you had the stroke, your symptoms and your speed of recovery will vary.

- You might want to check with your physical therapist to see if electric muscle stimulation would benefit you, especially if you are experiencing chronic muscle weakness in your leg.

- If you do use an electric muscle stimulator, your therapist might direct you to manually move your limb in rhythm with the on cycle and relax it in the off cycle.

- This works well if you apply the electrodes to the back of your thigh, stimulating the hamstrings, stand at a counter and lift your calf every time the contraction starts. This way you are training your muscle to react in real time.

- You know your body so well that you'll notice improvements in range of motion and strength.

- If you detect pain, use heat or ice, massage, or a pain-relief gel to relieve the area that hurts. You'll also be able to detect any new weakness.

- When you experience weakness, compensate by exercising specifically to strengthen that area, or ask your therapist about using electric muscle stimulation.

- You may find that some days you feel super strong and your range of movement is noticeably increased, yet the next day you notice more pain, more stiffness and lack of balance.

- Don't feel you're backsliding if you have an off day.

- Keep in mind that if you experience weakness, it may be related to the fact that you overdid it when you felt great.

- If you find that your leg is weak when you get up after sleeping, push the heel hard into the floor a few times and stiffen the leg. This will ignite the muscles and wake them up.

- If you expect your journey of stroke rehabilitation to be an perfectly upward linear path, you will be disappointed.

- Just as the stock market has little up and down blips, so will your recovery. It's important to realize that you are trending upward rather than constantly achieving daily progress.

- Don't let frustration get out of hand. Just as a baby doesn't learn to walk in a week, it will take time for you to regain your coordination and ambulatory capabilities. And you absolutely can.

- No matter how smart or educated you are, you need to face the fact that your body is in recovery mode. If you feel that you're too sophisticated to be wasting time on boring baby-steps, this will probably not help your speed of recovery.

- Even though you may feel at times that you're not progressing very quickly, steady improvement can be measurable when calculated at monthly or even weekly intervals.

- Becoming annoyed is not going to help you. Reality is that your body is weak and you are going to have to retrain it to do your bidding. You can win.

- Remember that the secret is regaining mobility through movement. Just do small steps—but a lot of them.

- Ask your physical therapist to regularly measure your grip strength, your range of motion in your wrist and shoulder, and your weight-bearing capacity.

- You'll feel more confident that you're making progress when you can see improvement reflected in range-of-motion measurements.

- There is a light at the end of the tunnel. Just because you can't see it yet doesn't mean that it's not there.

- Determination helps. Just keep heading towards your goal. You will actually find that at times progress comes faster than you anticipated.

- Progress will come in bursts. You may feel stagnant for a few days, and suddenly you are able to perform movements that were impossible the week before.

- On good days, try and go for a good walk. Make sure you wear shoes that are not loose, and support your feet. It's better to be safe than fashionable.

- When you walk, dress appropriately for the weather. You won't feel like going for a walk if you're uncomfortable.

- Focus on the idea that your body is the horse your mind rides on. It is definitely weakened right now and will need to recover. Accept this and realize that repetitive movement and frequent practice are the keys to full mobility.

- Remembering all the physical therapy homework you have been given can be difficult. So make a list. Don't try and do all the exercises in one session. You'll progress more quickly if you just do a few exercises at a time.

- Check your exercises off as you do them. You'll be surprised how much strength you can gain with just a few minutes of exercise sprinkled throughout your day.

- In order to improve your balance and strengthen your core, stand up straight and sit up straight. Your posture is an important component in increasing muscular strength and the accumulated effect of practicing good posture can be significant.

Avoiding Another Stroke

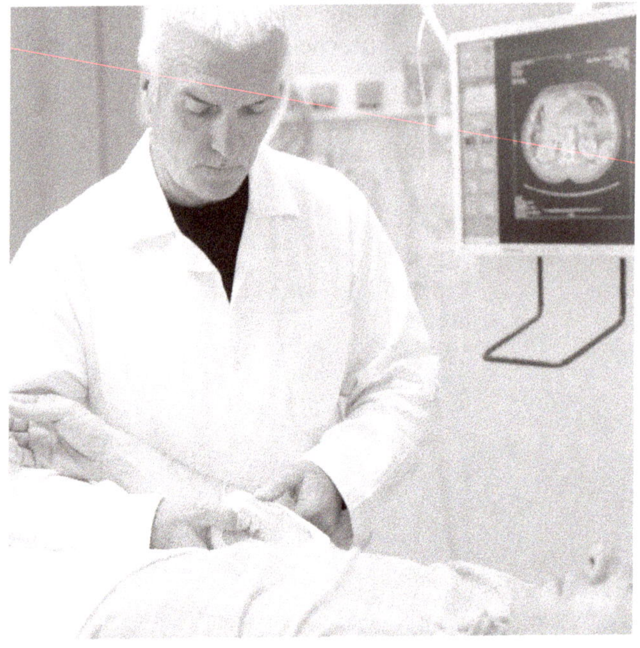

- With improved clot-busting drugs and other therapy, more people survive strokes today than ever before..

- Today we also know that taking prescribed medicines and instigating changes in lifestyle can dramatically reduce the risk of having a second stroke.[46]

- Stroke survivors are most vulnerable to second stroke risk during the first three months after a stroke. The risk of a having a second stroke remains a factor for up to five years after the first one.

- But you can prevent a second stroke. Studies show that with appropriate lifestyle changes, stroke victims can actually increase their life expectancy beyond that of the general population. [6]

- Post-stroke recovery can feel daunting, especially when the risk of a second stroke exists. But small lifestyle changes will stabilize your health. Being consistent is the best way to lower the chances of recurring health problems.

- Studies have shown the importance of controlling vascular risk factors to prevent the re-occurrence of a stroke. So be alert to signs of heightened blood pressure or diabetes. [46, 50]

- Stroke has a lot in common risk-wise, with diabetes, cardiovascular problems and hypertension. Today's sophisticated prescription medications can't "cure" you of these health problems, but they can definitely lower the risk of a second stroke. [46]

- High blood pressure is a leading cause of weakened arteries, since blood continuously pushes against the artery walls.

- Controlling your blood pressure is very important in terms of avoiding another stroke. [1, 3, 4] Treatment of elevated blood pressure reduces the risk of having a second stroke by 30%. [1]

- The most effective way to lower the risk of having a second stroke, is to focus on lowering your blood pressure to normal parameters. So measure your blood pressure often and ask your doctor's advice regarding keeping it in check. [46, 52]

- Many doctors recommend reducing cholesterol and stress levels wherever possible. So take your cholesterol-lowering meds and focus on relaxation.

- If your doctor has prescribed medicine to help you control your cholesterol, blood pressure, or diabetes, don't slack off or skip doses. Not taking your medicine is an important risk factor for repeat stroke.[46].

- It's common and often essential to seek guidance when managing the variety of prescribed medications during stroke recovery. Get help if you find it difficult to keep track of your meds.

- According to one study in patients with coronary artery disease, those patients who took 75 percent or less of their medications as prescribed had a four times higher risk of stroke than patients who took their medications exactly as directed.[46]

- Even if you're recovering well and you feel better, it's essential to keep high blood pressure, high blood cholesterol and diabetes under control by taking every pill you're prescribed every time and not discontinuing medications until your doctor gives you the go-ahead.[46]

- Complications that lead to diabetes are often also related to stroke, and so managing diet, exercise, and medications is a solid line of defense.

- As soon as possible, make it a point to get moving. Even minimal exercise is a good start. Physical activity will get your blood circulating and your lymphatic system moving.

- Its also important to get active. Harvard medical research recommends working out at least five times a week, even if the exercise is small and tailored to your capabilities.

- Up to 30 minutes of daily exercise is ideal, but exercise periods can be broken up if your schedule or ability level does not allow for such a long stretch.[46,51,52]

- Don't allow yourself to become distracted and forget to exercise. Attach a note to your bathroom mirror as a reminder.

- Once you start exercising, you will increase your neuroplasticity and muscle strength, and then find it easier every day to walk or do other light exercise.

- Immobility can become a habit, so make sure it doesn't.

- While continued care is recommended, it's not always given. So make sure you see your doctor regularly and arrange for regular physical therapy.

- Check with your doctor regarding any risks factors you have, such as atrial fibrillation which can lead to another stroke. The irregular heartbeat caused by atrial fibrillation is one of the leading causes of stroke and should be more closely monitored by your doctor during the recovery period.[46]

- Other risk factors, such as depression and obstructive sleep apnea, can also add to the risk of recurrent stroke. If you notice these symptoms, let your doctor know.

- A recently published study by Johns Hopkins and Yale University School of Medicine showed that stroke patients can likely prevent another occurrence by eating well.[53]

- A diet rich in fruit and vegetables has actually been associated with a 21 percent lower risk of stroke.

- Finding an ideal diet after a stroke can sometimes be difficult due to muscular or digestive issues. So focus on vibrant, bold, and simple foods—vegetables, fruit and lean meats. These can help lower cholesterol and inflammatory issues throughout your body.[53, 54]

- As well as eating a good plant-based diet, try to avoid processed foods, and make sure you have a good source of polyunsaturated fat, such as olive oil. [53]

- It's a good idea to try to slim down. Balancing calorie intake with exercise is an excellent first step.

- Keep an eye on your Body Mass Index. If you know your weight and height, you can figure out your BMI by googling "calculate BMI"

- If you still smoke, do whatever it takes to quit. Cutting out tobacco eases dangerous stress on the blood vessels in your brain, heart and elsewhere.

- Smoking restricts oxygen in the blood, leading to complications that can cause another stroke, as well as respiratory illnesses.

- The risk of stroke doubles in smokers compared to non-smokers, so focusing on cutting this habit should be a priority moving forward. [52,53]

-

- Avoid becoming stressed out, since this will probably send hormones such as adrenaline and cortisol racing through your system, raising your blood pressure in the process.

- Make it a point to relax as much as possible, and when frustration arises, try to deal with it in a relaxed way. Calming activities including creative hobbies, yoga and meditation can be helpful..

- Major stroke centers also recommend minimizing alcohol consumption because alcohol can raise your blood pressure. It's advisable have no more than two drinks per day. Anything more can increase the risk of stroke by 50%. [52, 53]

Communicating with Your Doctor

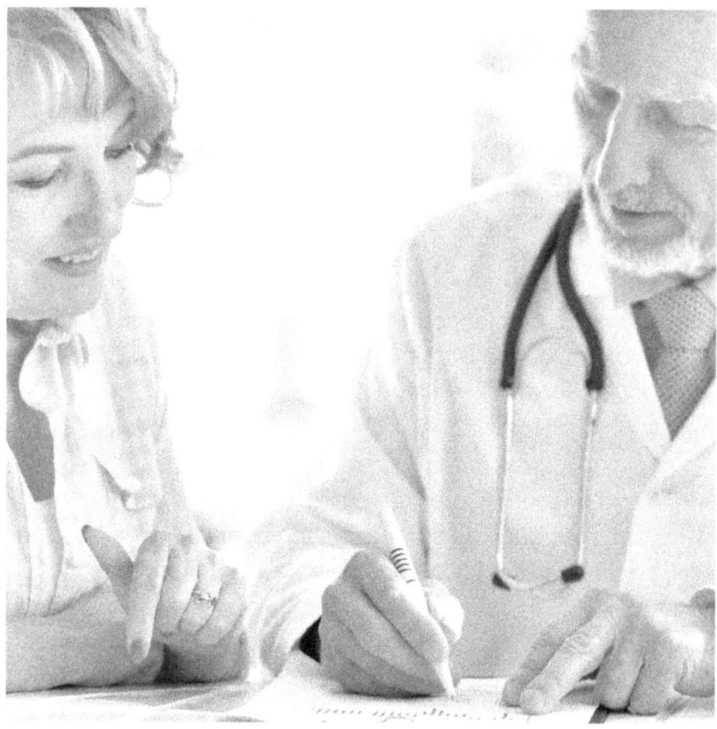

- Go to your doctor as soon as you are released from the hospital and get written permission for a handicapped parking placard.

- If you need a wheelchair, you might want to purchase one that is light weight, so it's easy to put it in and out of the car. Check with your insurance company or Medicare to see if it will be covered.

- See your doctor regularly and have blood work done every 3 months. Treatment often focuses on the first three months after a stroke, but patients need to be followed long-term.[46]

- Monitoring your blood pressure is important in keeping your blood pressure within healthy limits. Talk to your doctor about controlling your blood pressure. He or she may recommend medication.

- Even if you are not diagnosed with high blood pressure, have your blood pressure checked regularly.

- The risk of high blood pressure is greater if you're older than age 35, overweight or a smoker.

- Factors that can help lower blood pressure include increasing exercise (a daily walk is beneficial), managing your stress, cutting back on caffeine, quitting smoking, and limiting alcohol.

- If you are diabetic, talk to your doctor about controlling your blood glucose. Diabetes is definitely a risk factor for stroke because it damages the inner lining of arteries and makes it easier for plaque and clots to attach.

- Even if you are on insulin, keep your eye on your blood glucose levels. Also cool it with refined sugars and starches, instead eat plenty of good quality protein and green vegetables.

- Keep in mind that one refined carb binge can send your glucose level into the stratosphere. Measure your blood glucose morning and night and try to keep it within healthy limits.

- Take your medications as prescribed and don't skip doses. It's easier to remember to take your meds if you take them at the same time each day.

- If you haven't had your eyes checked since your stroke, have an eye examination. Many stroke survivors have affected vision and your optical prescription may need to be adjusted.

- You may have difficulty noticing objects outside the central field of vision on your affected side. You don't want to bump into an object because you didn't notice it.

- If you have trouble focusing your eyes since your stroke, let your doctor and physical or occupational therapist know. There are specific eye exercises which are effective in restoring focus.

- Common complications of stroke include swelling of the brain, swallowing problems that can lead to pneumonia, and urinary tract infections. If you notice any symptoms, see your doctor immediately.

- Check with your doctor, your insurance company, your physical therapist or Medicare to see how much insurance coverage you have.

- When it comes to hospital and outpatient rehabilitation therapy, there is a wide range of coverage from one insurance company to another. You don't want any expensive surprises.

- If you are denied coverage for physical or occupational therapy on the basis of lack of medical necessity, be aware that your doctor can go to bat for you, appeal the insurance company's decision and forward them a copy of your medical records.

- You can also call your insurance company and appeal a decision.

- Realize that you have a right to all your medical records, including hospital records, brain image films, and physical therapy notes.

- It's probably a good idea to have a copy of your medical records, especially if you are applying for disability benefits.

- If you notice a decline in your self-care, motor or speech abilities, be sure to alert your doctor. You may be eligible for more rehabilitation therapy services from Medicare.

- Your doctor will probably give you an Advanced Health-Care Directive form. Since you've had one brush with death, it's probably advisable for you and your spouse to each fill one out.

- An Advanced Health-Care Directive lays out instructions for treatment when you reach the end stage.

- Another useful form is a specific type of power of attorney or health care proxy, in which you can authorize someone to make decisions on your behalf if and when you might be incapacitated.

- Community resources, such as stroke survivor and caregiver support groups, are available for you and for your caregiver. Your doctor can refer you to a social worker who can help you find resources in your community.

Getting Relief from Pain

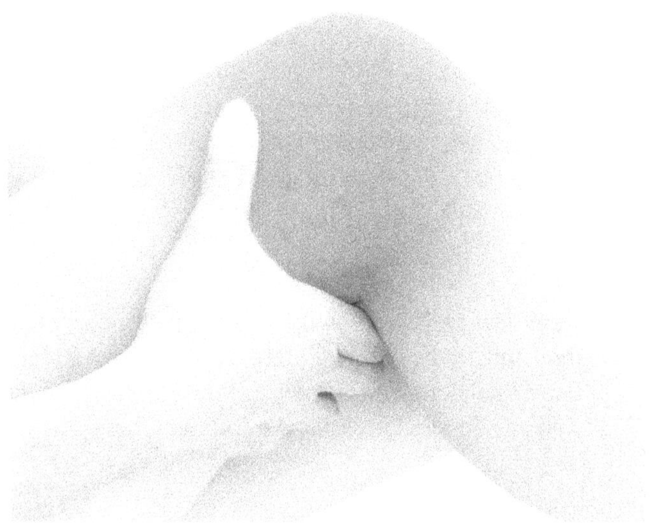

- Pain can obviously interfere with your functionality, sleep, moods and outlook

- Pain is so personal that only you know how uncomfortable and disruptive your pain is. It is invisible to others..

- Keep in mind that your stronger arm is going to get a work out. So be aware of this, especially when using your wheelchair and when getting out of bed.

- If you don't give your strong arm a rest it will become sore and that's not going to help since you're depending on it.

- Use medication when necessary but also realize that pain is a kind of feedback and if you block it out with pain-killers, you might damage your muscles by unknowingly performing tasks that are outside the range of your capacity.

- If you are willing to forgo medication, consider that heat can relieve muscle pain and so can ice cold. Some therapists recommend applying heat and cold alternatively, especially when muscles are in spasm.

- Keep yourself as comfortable as you can. Do you need pain medication? Are you trying to do too much? Do you simply need to distract yourself by watching a good movie and deal with any issues later? Remember, you have lots of time.

Strengthening a Weak Leg

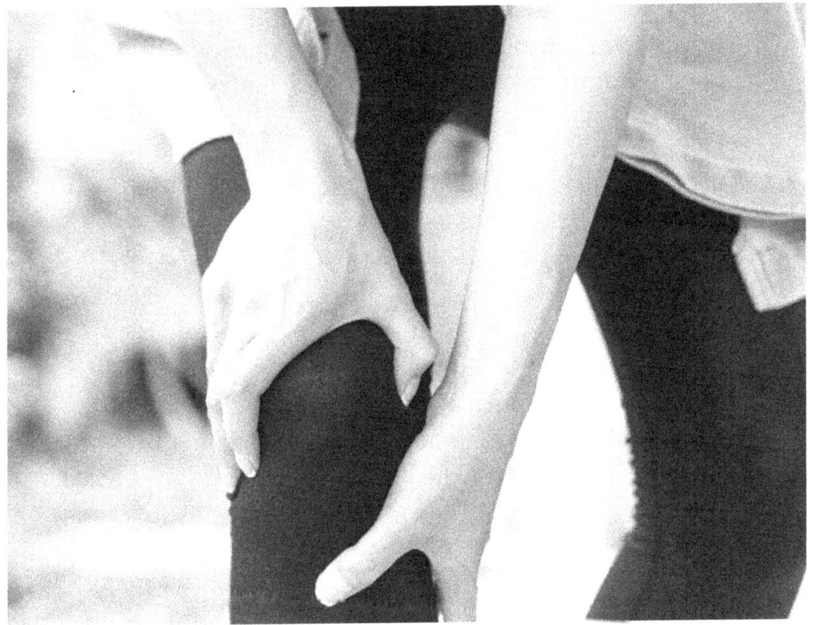

- Leg muscle weakness is one of the biggest risk factors for falls.

- A weak leg will definitely increase the danger of falling. Do your leg strengthening exercises. You'll be safer.

- You will help your weak leg become stronger by putting all your weight on that leg when you get up from a sitting position— using a cane or prop for balance.

- You can increase the strength of your weak leg by supporting yourself with a cane and putting your weight on your weak leg when you're getting up from a sitting position.

- Most stroke patients tend to put their weight on their strong leg but this doesn't help strengthen the leg that needs it.

- It's a good idea to do a few squats with your weight on your weak leg and also do some lunges, putting your weight on your weak leg but making sure you don't let your knee go past your toes.

- You can also strengthen your weak leg by using a plastic squishy 6" plastic ball. Sit on the floor or in bed. Push the ball under your weak knee into the floor or mattress, and hold it down for 10 seconds. Then relax for 10 seconds. This will strengthen the muscles that hold you up.

- Do the same exercise upright, pushing the ball behind your weak knee against a wall for 8-10 seconds.

- While anchoring yourself with a stable support such as a counter or sink, repeatedly stand on your tip toes and then your heels to strengthen the muscles you use for walking. Do 10 reps a couple times per day.

- Knee bends are good because they will improve your ability to stand up after sitting. Doing side steps along the kitchen counter will help with balance and coordination.

- One easy technique for strengthening your leg when you stand up is to push the heel of your weak leg hard into the floor. Stiffen your leg. This weight-bearing exercise will aid proprioception — your body's sense of the position and motion of your joints.

- Proprioception encourages involuntary reflexes to stabilize and protect you by maintaining posture and balance when you move. This is especially vital for joints like the knee. Proprioception is a significant factor in balance, graceful movement and injury prevention

Predictable Psychological Changes

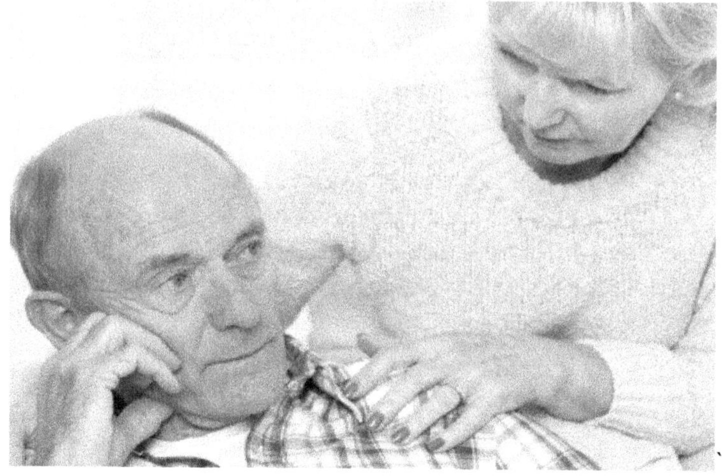

- After having had a stroke, you will probably experience emotional and behavioral changes.

- This is because our brain controls our behavior, emotions, logical thought and insight.

- Patients describe many reactions to their experience of having a stroke. Some find it quite frightening or bewildering. Some cannot remember having the stroke, or even being ill, and these gaps in memory can be confusing.

- Understanding the emotional impact of having a stroke will help you work through what has happened. Assessment is crucial and will benefit you from the outset of having the stroke to the longer term.

- Since stroke happens suddenly and without warning, virtually all stroke survivors have had no preparation whatsoever for psychological symptoms. All of a sudden your emotional world can be turned upside down.

- Some people have very vivid memories of treatment procedures, which may also be troubling. Others may seem to cope better but are still obviously upset that they have suffered a stroke.

- Your psychological health is as important as your physical recovery, and your mood can actually enhance or deter how quickly you recover.

- Since your mind can focus on only one thing at a time, replace the downward spiral of negativity with personal encouragement and positive expectation.

- Use mantras such as "I am feeling stronger" and "I am recovering well" to crowd out doubt, and the feeling that you may be at a standstill.

- Understanding and patience will help a lot. You are likely to drop things, lose track of items and have more spills because of the cognitive effects of the stroke.

- Realize that your capacity for multi-tasking is more limited than it was pre-stroke and accept this as the new reality rather than getting frustrated.

- Discipline can disappear when you arrive home after a stroke. Once you get home from the hospital there is no external source forcing or even encouraging you.

- Make sure to make your bed, get dressed, shower, focus on your grooming, eat nutritious food, keep your space tidy, go for your daily walk and do your physical therapy routine.

- Try to pick up after yourself and stay organized, otherwise you'll tend to constantly lose or misplace things, and this can be very frustrating, since it will take longer to get things done.

- Set up a system where everything has its place. Be observant and pay more attention to what you're doing in order to avoid having to constantly pick up dropped items, clean up spills or search for missing items.

- You'll also find it helpful to make a "to do" list of basic daily tasks and follow it. Each time you cross off a completed task, you'll have a sense of accomplishment.

- It's important to be alert to possible behavioral changes, especially if you perceive others acting "differently" to you.

- Depending on what part of your brain the stroke has affected, you may have a range of symptoms, including slow thinking, poor reasoning, memory loss (especially short term memory), being more accident prone and experiencing unpredictable emotional behavior. Your insight may also be affected.

- Injury from a stroke may make you careless, irritable or confused. You may also feel anxiety, anger and suffer mood swings.

- Depending on how seriously you are impacted physically, your self-esteem may be affected.

- If your stroke impacted the part of your brain that controls your emotions, you may perceive own behavior as pretty much the same as it was before the stroke, and you may not notice that you are acting any differently. But others may.

- Consider the possibility that you may have experienced changes in cognition and memory. For example, you may repeat yourself often. You may be constantly misplacing things.

- It's best not to assume others will clean up your messes. Try to remember to clean up after yourself.

- It's important to pay attention. If you cut yourself peeling an apple when you're taking a blood thinner, it can be messy.

- Try to be as focused as you can. Make lists. Compensate for your symptoms by actively paying attention. You'll become considerably more efficient as time passes.

- Your memory may be affected So make a list of things you'll want to leave in your car. Sunglasses, reading glasses, a shopping bag, a pen, a checkbook and credit card, your cane, a water bottle, your handicapped parking placard, even floss sticks can be handy when you need them.

- Always bring your cell phone, your tablet, a snack, paper towels and your shopping list with you when you leave the house.

- You may find that you may often unconsciously focus on the losses that the stroke has presented you with, while at other times you may focus on the process of restoring your life.

- Your mind is analyzing and processing both the good and the bad: grieving the things you have lost, while focusing on re-building what you can to re-establish normalcy.

- Stay positive by screening your thoughts. Set up a mental filter. Avoid negative people, turn off TV stations that feature argumentative talk. Think of the best things about your life.

- Try to be a positive influence on everyone you interact with. Make a list of everything you are grateful for. Know that you will recover better than ever if you maintain an unshakable belief in a great future.

- Don't be afraid to be wrong. You're learning a new way of functioning and sometimes you have to let go of your ego.

- Occasionally your therapist will suggest ideas that you feel underestimate your capabilities, are extra cautious, and are potentially a waste of time. But don't be resistant. You need to accept these suggestions and keep improving.

- Research has shown that stroke patients who had a right brain stroke tend to become more impatient, less insightful and interrupt often. They also tend to get things out of sequence or misinterpret or confuse information.

- A stroke affecting the left brain may cause speech problems and a slowing down of thought and reactions. [1, 25]

- To get yourself on solid psychological ground it is important for you to spend a little time doing an analysis of your condition and figure out where you're at physically, mentally and emotionally.

- A professional psychological evaluation can be beneficial. Psychologists have found that the initial acute stage of disorientation is followed by insecurity and anger, followed by the struggle between hope for recovery and the reality of lost capacity.

- Reactions to stroke differ widely. Some people seem to adjust well to being hospitalized, but feel anxious when they go home. Others remain mildly disoriented.

- We go through a series of emotional stages in order to adjust and normalize our psychological reactions to stroke as we recover.

- Psychologists liken the stages most stroke patients go through, to the four stages of grief after bereavement: shock and numbness; acute distress (anxiety and anger); grief and mourning (depression) and the final stage of adjusting to and accepting the new reality.

- Fear is an inevitable side-effect of a stroke, but it can interfere with your ability to make appropriate choices. You are probably a lot more capable than you realize.

- If you are so fearful that you are hesitant to push yourself hard enough to get those muscles moving again, you'll stall your progress.

- Figure out the dividing line between being overly fearful and taking risks. Risky behavior can result in a fall, but on the other hand, you need to become active.

- If you're rendered dysfunctional by the fear of dying, you're not really living. Don't give up the chance to enjoy your remaining years by giving in to fear.

- Fear is basically protective, but when fear is dominating your life, it's time to deal with it. Try to face up to your fears.

- Figure out what's the worst that can happen. Probably dying. It happens to everyone and it will happen to you at some point. So make a commitment to focus on enjoying all the life you have left.

- Distract yourself from your fear by putting energy into your life and visualizing success. You'll be able to will spend time with your family, become more mobile, enjoy lots of great conversations, beautiful scenery, stunning sunsets and other wonderful experiences.

- Talk to your physical therapist about your fears and he or she will give you guidelines for the most appropriate course of action based on your present capability. Some of your fears may be baseless.

- If your therapist says "You can do it!" He or she knows you can, so repeat this phrase as a mantra and plunge on ahead. Remember, the time you can most impact your life is right now.

- Physical therapists report that many stroke patients become loud and uncooperative when they are assisting with exercises that cause the patient discomfort or even minor pain. You may be in your 60's or 70's and your therapists may be in their 20's but that doesn't mean they don't know what they're doing.

- Sometimes physical therapy may feel a bit uncomfortable, but it's necessary. You'll advance a lot faster by being cooperative.

- When you are dismissive, oppositional or uncooperative, you're not giving your physical therapists the positive reinforcement that can motivate their therapy most effectively.

- Your therapists are committed to helping others and they probably dislike being unappreciated or talked down to.

- Consider that your therapist has scientific knowledge and familiarity with techniques that can help you recover. This expertise is critical in helping you to regain the use of your weak side.

- You might have access to counseling or be able to participate in a support group. Counseling and group support can help you improve impaired cognitive abilities, such as memory, processing, problem-solving, social skills, judgment and safety awareness.

- Therapy for communication disorders is also important. Speech therapy can help you regain lost abilities in speaking, listening, writing and comprehension.

- Trust is a huge issue for stroke patients. Your nurses, doctors and physical therapists are all telling you it will get easier and you'll get better as time passes. But at the same time, you are very aware that you are absent-minded, insecure and anxious, that one side of your body is dysfunctional, and that you need mobility aids.

- Are your healthcare professionals just being encouraging to make you feel better? Actually no. One thing you can count on is that there are measurable and established physical and emotional recovery stages post-stroke and the emotional stages coordinate with your physical rehabilitation.

- You may notice that your nervous system is hyper-alert and that you startle easily. Your nervous system has been attacked and is in PTSD mode, protecting itself from any more nasty surprises.

- Make it a point to try and relax, steer clear of drama, watch the news less often, limit your exposure to negative or oppositional people and try to sail through this period with calmness and equanimity.

- If you are feeling discouraged or experiencing a setback, act as your own counselor. Speak quietly to yourself. Give yourself encouragement. Console yourself as a friend would.

- Guide yourself through discouragement. You've managed to steer yourself through challenging periods in the past and you can do it now.

- Circumstances can't weaken you, unless you let them. Dealing with adversity will strengthen you. Once you've managed to succeed, you'll know you can always do it from here on out.

- If you constantly complain and make excuses for not following through on exercising, eating well and doing your physical therapy, no one would deny that you have the right to take that position.

- You do have a great excuse for not feeling motivated. But in reality, movement is a crucial component of stroke recovery.

- Avoid being a demanding pain in the neck. Yes life is unfair. Yes you didn't anticipate having a stroke. Yes it's easy to feel sorry for yourself. But whether you accept it or not, genetics aside, your habitual patterns of behavior were probably complicit in causing your stroke.

- Remember that your mental and emotional experience is really up to you. Happiness is your choice. Enthusiasm for life is your choice. Being empathetic to others is your choice. Giving to others is your choice. Being positive is your choice.

- Whatever choices you make will highly affect your recovery and how you spend the rest of your life. When you become frustrated and angry, try to handle the issue in a way that causes less dissension. Calmness and kindness can become habits that make your life more agreeable.

Extreme Risk! How To Avoid A Fall

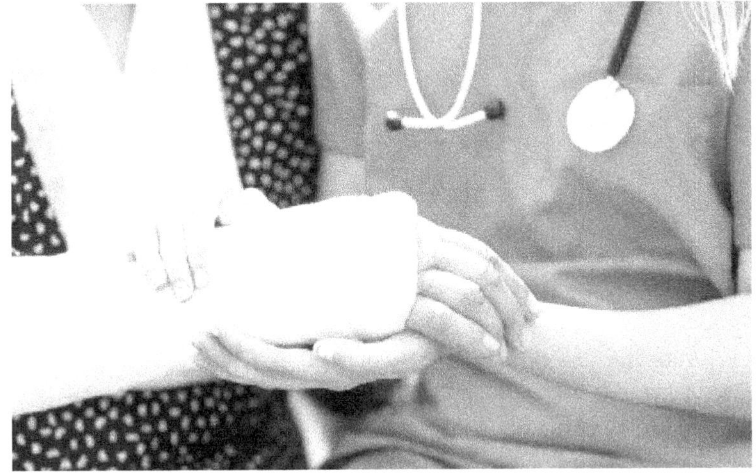

- Be aware of the danger of falling. A fall could cause injuries you may not think are serious, but may cause bruising or bleeding, especially if you are taking blood thinners.

- If you fall more than twice in 6 months, let your doctor or physical therapist know.

- Falling is actually the leading cause of accidental home deaths in stroke patients. So be careful. Be conservative, and avoid being overconfident. [12,13]

- Stroke patients have a higher likelihood of problems that make them more likely to fall. These problems range from dizziness to problems with balance, loss of vision, overall poor health and more. [12,13,14]

- People who have fallen in the past year are more likely to fall again. This is due in part to changes in their habits and activity level as a result of the first fall. [12,13,14]

- Falls are listed as a major reason for 40% of nursing home admissions. Falls can cause broken bones, increased disability, even death. [12,13,14]

- Studies have shown that stroke survivors are twice as likely to fall following a stroke and more than three times as likely as the general population to fall multiple times. [12,13,14]

- A recent 12-month follow-up study of first time stroke patients found that they had significantly lower scores on balance, mobility and balance confidence than the control group of non-stroke older adults, and fell 70% more often. Injuries ranged from fractures, bruising and sprains to cuts and scrapes. [14]

- If a stroke patient has brittle, thin bones due to osteoporosis, a fall can result in serious injury and even more problems with movement and getting around. [11]

- Stroke survivors recently discharged from rehabilitation facilities are almost twice as likely to experience falls than non-stroke older adults. Almost 50% of falls occur during the first month after the stroke. [12,13]

- Realize that it is not just your stroke that is increasing your risk of falling. If your other health problems such as diabetes, depression or arthritis aren't treated properly, you are more likely to fall. [12,13,14,15]

- Inactivity alone can put you at risk of falls, so make sure you find ways to become active and stay involved. [12,13,14,15]

- One little known factor in post-stroke falls, is that cognitive and memory problems also increase the risk of falls. Also, inactivity can cause a decline in your thinking abilities. [12,13,14]

- Let your doctor know if you feel you are not as sharp as you were before the stroke. He can refer you to a home care agency with staff whose main job is to help you stay safe in your home.

- If you do experience a fall, realize that you will probably have psychological consequences as well as bruises.

- You may experience typical symptoms of post-traumatic stress syndrome, including reliving the fall (especially as you are going to sleep), heightened anxiety about falling, balance insecurity, enhanced startle responses and a feeling of general over-stress. This is a normal protective reaction.

- If you do experience anxiety after a fall, try to avoid getting stressed out about being stressed out. Relax, learn from the experience and make a vow to pay attention so that you don't fall again.

- Most falls occurred among patients who had reduced muscular tone (70%), paralysis (54%) and numbness in the weak side of the body. [14]

- To cut the risk of falling, be aware of potential hazards. Focus on really paying attention to where you are in relation to your immediate environment.

- Look for things you could trip on or bump into. If you stub your toe on the weak side your tendency will be to fall in that direction. If your sight is affected on one side, scan the field of view on that affected side often. With practice, you'll get a lot better at noticing the entire field of vision.

- If you feel like this doesn't apply to you, realize that you are really not immune no matter how well you're progressing. You are indeed quite vulnerable and need to take care. Most falls for stroke patients occur while walking, doing transfers or bathing. Remember, one moment of inattention can hurt you. Really.

- Pushing yourself beyond your comfort zone increases risk. If you press past your comfort limits, you'll get tired, sloppy and become more accident prone.

- If you push yourself, every time you overdo it, you'll feel even more exhausted. The mantra is: "Things take time!"

- If you are progressing well, be careful about overestimating your ability in terms of physical activity.

- You may feel energetic and want to just keep going, but when you exert yourself too much, you run the risk of getting sloppy, making a misjudgment and falling.

- Making great progress with mobility can actually increase the opportunities for falling. So try to avoid becoming over-confident.

- There are effective precautions you can use to decrease your chances of falling. First, don't be in a hurry. Multitasking is a no no.

- Slow down to reduce your risk of making mistakes. Most important, make sure you use your cane or walker even at home. You don't win any awards for walking unaided, especially if you fall. Falling is a F grade in stroke rehab.

- If you experience dizziness, it's important to let your doctor know. There are many causes of dizziness, including side effects of medicine, dehydration, dietary problems, high blood pressure, or visual problems caused by your stroke. Dizziness can also be caused by stroke damage to certain areas of the brain.

- Your dizziness may be related to your medications, especially if two medicines interact with each other. Have your doctor review all your medicines with you, to avoid undesired interactions.

- A recent study showed that in a significant percentage of falls, stroke patients were found to be using hypoglycemic, antihypertensive, tranquilizing or neuroleptic drugs. [14] So it's important to get your doctor to investigate whether your medications may put you at risk.

- One often overlooked cause of dizziness is postural hypotension which occurs when your blood pressure drops significantly when you sit up from lying down or stand up from sitting. Getting up quickly can rob your brain of blood flow and cause you to feel dizzy or faint.

- To compensate for postural hypotension, you can make it a habit of slowly counting to five while rising from one position to the next. This gives your heart time to adjust to pumping blood against gravity.

- Be aware that certain medications can be a factor in postural hypotension so let your doctor know if you experience dizziness when getting up.

Maintaining Motivation

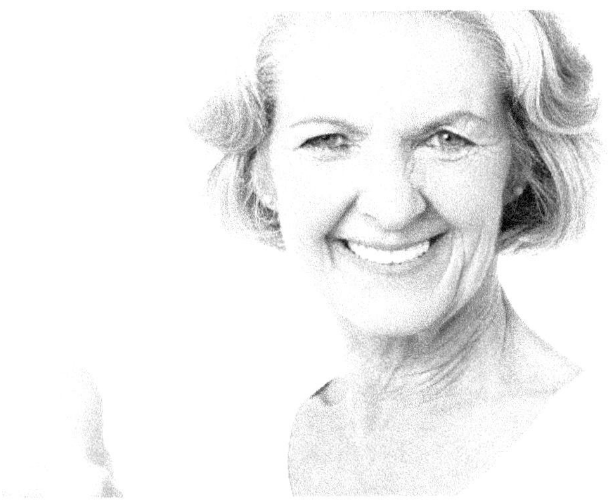

- Of all the hints, hacks, strategies, advice and shortcuts you will encounter in your stroke recovery, by far the most important factor is how motivated you are.

- On one hand you have motivation, inspiration and positive reinforcement, on the other hand you have doubt, insecurity, depression, fear, distraction and lack of hope. It's up to you to choose your path.

- How motivated are you? If you're highly motivated, you'll embrace rehab and recover faster than someone who is satisfied with letting their body recover automatically and at its own speed.

- Keep in mind that those who recover the fastest from a stroke are the most highly motivated. They refuse to believe that they will be disabled for a long time and recover quickly.

- Use visualization as a tool for healing. Imagine your nerves becoming active and your muscles building gradually cell-by-cell as you become stronger and more capable.

- Healing will become automatic to a certain extent if you set the process into motion with mental oversight and reinforce it with your physical therapy exercises. Every repetition brings you closer to full functionality.

- Keep your attention on the fact that you are healing, that you are a good person, and that you deserve a good life. You'll find that a positive attitude will help the rehabilitation process.

- Try to be as objective as you can about your condition. Don't become swept up in the drama of playing the demanding victim. Observe yourself as would a person who doesn't know you. Are you overdoing the victim role?

- You are strong enough to have survived a stroke. Now your goal is complete rehabilitation. Yes, there will be frustrating days. Yes, you will be disabled while you are recovering, but you can definitely get back your strength and your control.

- Avoid naysayers. Everyone knows someone who was severely impacted by a stroke. That doesn't mean you can't fully recover.

- Remember that your relatives and friends are actually trying to help you when they tell you about Uncle Jimmy who never got better. They want to protect you from disappointment.

- Your best defense to peoples' "helpful" stories of failure is to remain detached. Regard this kind of information as irrelevant.

- Ignore the "what if's" and the "if only's." Your confidence is more powerful. Remember you are a unique case study of one. It's up to you.

- The stroke happened to you and you only, not to the friends and relatives who are giving you their opinions and advice. It's important that you live your life for yourself, and fulfil your own dreams and expectations rather than the opinions and expectations of others.

- Keep in mind that boredom can be counter-productive. It's fairly easy to get bogged down and overwhelmed unless you are motivated, especially when you don't have the schedule imposed by working at a regular job.

- Remember that real change can be difficult at the beginning. Life after a stroke is a new existence. Without the familiar to rely upon, you may not feel as much in control as you may have been in the past.

- When things are not going your way, you may start doubting yourself. But if you stay motivated, positive, and keep moving in the direction of healing, your breakthrough will happen and you will be on a fast track to recovery.

- Consider that you will have times when you feel discouraged, The reality of your situation, however, is that you don't really have a choice but to push through the discouragement and do whatever it takes to recover. You can do it.

- Try to do something new and challenging every day, especially if you spend your days at home. Call old friends you haven't seen for a while and spend time on hobbies such as playing cards, which help you stretch your memory and give you a social outlet.

- Prepare a dish from a new recipe. Do crosswords. Read an exciting best-seller. Play cards or play Scrabble, Sudoku or Words With Friends which you can do online.

- Divide your goals into short-term, medium-range and long term goals. What activities are you going to do in the next three days to help you get stronger?

- A daily walk is good. Make a list and follow through. What will you be able to accomplish a month from now? Six months from now? How will you reward yourself when you accomplish these goals? Write your daily goals as tasks on your "To Do" list.

- Predicting your own recovery speed can be difficult. Some people do really well for the first four or five months, then they stop doing their rehab exercises and level off. Others never level off, and have a continuous upward curve.

- The secret to continued progress, is to avoid leveling off on your rehab exercises, so do whatever helps to stay motivated and keep at it.

- People who are able to fully recover from a stroke have been motivated enough to seriously apply themselves, practice repetitive movement and learn basic motor skills again. You can too. It will pay you to work hard and get with the program.

- It may be difficult to get going, especially if you're feeling isolated or depressed, but you'll do so much better if you focus on making positive changes rather than going the self-pity route.

- Do a self-evaluation. Figure out what are your strengths.

- Where does it hurt? How strong is your affected leg? How moveable is your shoulder? Your hand? Your wrist? How well can you straighten your fingers? Separate them? Make a fist?

- How confident do you feel? Are you sad? Are you impatient or irritable? Once you figure out where you're at, you'll have a solid basis for behaving appropriately and feel more secure in handling situations as they arise.

- There is a wide range of recovery speeds in stroke victims. The common factor in those who heal the fastest, is a stubborn positivity. Erase "I can't" from your thoughts. Frustration won't help.

- The most important aspect of stroke recovery, is encapsulated in the words of Winston Churchill. He said "never give in, never give in, never, never, never, never." Believe in yourself and your ability to heal. You will have to practice hundreds of repetitions, but you can do it.

- Positivity, confidence and persistence are the three factors which will enable you to overcome the symptoms your stroke has caused. Stay positive, so that you will avoid depression. Be confident, knowing others have achieved complete recovery. And persist, so you won't backslide.

- It's up to you to keep yourself motivated and entertained. Any activities that you can participate in that will build up your confidence are good. If you like to sing, turn on the radio or a music app, select an oldies station and join in with the music. You know the words. Go for it.

- If you can stand, let yourself move to dance music, even if you have to hang on to a counter or heavy table. Any exercise you can do is great. And if it has rhythm, all the better.

- One thing to consider is that you are in the autumn of your life. You don't have to run around after little kids any more, you are wiser, probably more spiritually inclined. Your days of serious production and workaholism are over.

- Enjoy this time. You can now relax, see more sunsets, watch your grandkids growing up and not have the responsibility of raising them.

- It's important to focus on grooming. Shower daily and use a skin brush. Have your hair cut or styled regularly. Ladies put on your makeup, even if merely going to physical therapy. Wear an outfit that complements you.

- People will respond to you positively when you look stylish and upbeat. It seems that people will respect you more when it's obvious that you respect yourself.

- Staying highly motivated involves focusing on the most effective and proven systems for increasing your personal drive to succeed.

- Of course, everyone is different, but one characteristic we all have in common is that we will work for a reward. So set yourself goals.

- Reward yourself when you stay on schedule, practice good form in your exercise routine and extend your range of motion. Make a list of things you like to do, such as watching good movies, going to the park, having lunch with a friend. Choose a reward from your list when you're doing well.

- Doubt and lack of confidence can be insidious. Doubt can wreck your progress almost as severely as an injury.

- You can actually treat your stroke recovery like a job, your compensation being full recovery. How much would you pay if you could wave a magic wand and be completely recovered in a year? Well that's the equivalent of what your "earnings" will be when you accomplish a full recovery through your own efforts.

- Instead of getting frustrated with your body for not being as capable and efficient as it was pre-stroke, take the attitude of loving and respecting your body as part of loving and respecting yourself.

- Despite the limitations caused by your stroke, you are still the master of your fate and controller of your destiny. Keep in mind that you have the ability to heal, reconnect and reactivate your nerves and muscles.

- Treat yourself well. Feed yourself with nutritious meals. Exercise productively. Train your body to become functional again as you would an injured pet whom you love.

- Seeing your body as the enemy is not going to help you recover. Your body is an integral part of you. Remember, the limits you place on yourself can significantly affect your recovery.

- When you look back on your life, you'll probably find that the times you most remember are the times when you were challenged and you succeeded.

- Overcoming life's storms makes you stronger and the adventures you remember as being enjoyable were also probably rather challenging. You have risen to the occasion many times in your life and you can do it now.

- Remember that progress happens one tiny step at a time. Just keep at it. Doubt and pessimism will impede your progress. Stay positive, visualize healing, set goals you'll achieve when you recover, and let hope carry you forward.

- Focus on now and the task ahead. A mind that is constantly focused on the past is wasting brain power.

- Even though you may feel fragile, use this time to read and gather knowledge. Indulge yourself. Read the books and articles you've always been meaning to. Watch great movies on Netflix and Amazon. Email or write cards to your friends.

- Day by day, movement by movement, your strength will begin to return. The darkness will begin to clear, your appetite for life will begin to increase and you will spread your mental and emotional wings and fly into your future.

- You're different now. You've survived a crisis. Now you'll be able to calmly handle whatever life throws at you.

- It's important to focus on what's right with your progress rather than your limitations.

- Think about where you were at a month ago. Notice the improvements you have made. You are stronger now. You have more flexibility. The therapy is working. You are on a path to recovery.

- Obviously if you are a highly functional individual, doing something as boring as repetitive movements will come second to using your iPad, watching Netflix, or messaging your friends.

- You have to take control. There is really no alternate if you want to regain full function. Set a schedule to do your physical therapy and keep it.

Recognizing and Preventing Depression

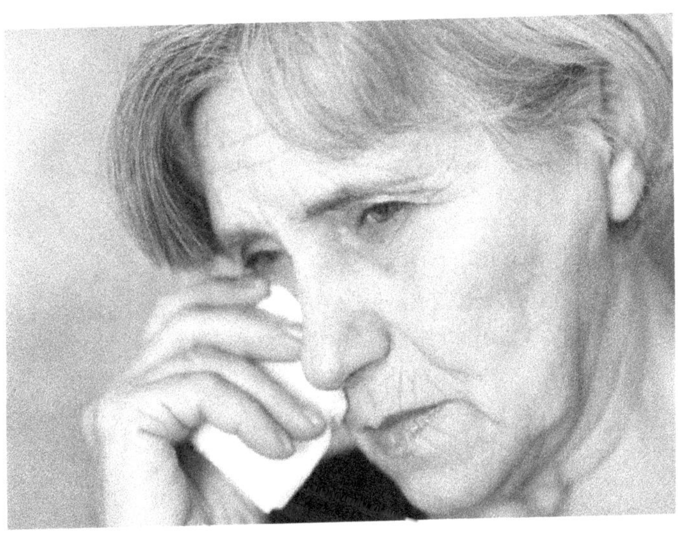

- Statistics show that fully one third of those who have had a stroke experience depression and 30% experience apathy.[15]

- Post stroke depression can actually interfere with your recovery. If you start feeling hopeless, discouraged, sad, anxious or worthless, it's time to get help.

- Many patients don't recognize depression or treat it. Why? Because people assume that "it's natural" to feel depressed or experience apathy after a stroke. Wrong! These conditions are effectively treatable.

- Post-stroke depression can result from biochemical changes in the brain resulting from the stroke; the impact of sudden losses in lifestyle; or a faulty thought-pattern, like a buggy computer program. What's more, your injured brain can having difficulty in processing positive emotions.

- Post stroke depression can actually interfere with your recovery. If you start feeling hopeless, discouraged, sad, anxious or worthless, it's time to get help. See your doctor as soon as you suspect that you may be depressed.

- If you find that you are depressed, have difficulty controlling your emotions, or if your caregiver notices changes in your emotional outlook or attitude, speak to your doctor about developing a treatment strategy.

- Depression is a medical condition. Your doctor has access to a wide variety of effective antidepressants so let medical science take the edge off.

- Depression can be insidious. You may find that you tend to experience universal thinking. Thoughts such as "I'll never be the same" are counter-productive. Words like "always, never, over, broken" are not helping your healing process.

- You'll feel a lot better if you keep your thoughts in the present, rather than bemoaning the fact that things are no longer the way they used to be pre-stroke. You can't change the past. It's gone. Second guessing won't help you.

- If any of your friends, coworkers, relatives or caregivers alert you to the possibility that you may be suffering with depression, don't be defensive. Share your thoughts and attitudes. They may be able to perceive something you haven't detected.

- If you are depressed, your doctor may refer you to a psychologist. Cognitive behavior therapy has common ground with neuroscience and has been found by many patients to be as effective as taking anti-depressants.[16]

- Cognitive psychologists believe that patients' emotions, behaviors and physiology are influenced by their thoughts, and that it is not the situation itself that determines what patients feel but rather how they interpret the situation.[16]

- Stroke patients who receive cognitive behavior therapy often end up better, wiser, more empathetic and even more physically functional after their rehab is completed, than patients relying solely on medication.[16]

- If you are not into taking pharmaceutical medications you may want to take niacinamide as a supplement to help with depression. It has been found to be quite effective in treating depression and increasing energy.[17] Niacin is one of the B vitamins, but unless it is in the amide form, it can cause uncomfortable flushing with a prickly feeling in the skin, so make sure you use niacinamide rather than niacin. It is not toxic. Since it is a water-soluble vitamin you will pee out any excess.

- Another natural way to combat depression is saffron. A double blind, randomized trial tested saffron versus Prozac. For six weeks, 40 outpatients diagnosed with clinical depression got capsules containing 30 mg of the spice saffron—or, identical-looking capsules, containing 20 mg of Prozac.

- The results of the saffron vs Prozac study showed that within just one week, there was a significant drop in depression symptoms, and symptoms improved throughout the six weeks. The Prozac group and the saffron group reported similar results. However, whereas 20% percent of the Prozac users reported experiencing sexual dysfunction—a common side effect— not one did in the saffron group. So evidence indicates saffron may be a valuable alternate strategy. [18, 19]

- Whether or not you feel depressed, you should make an effort to maintain a social support network. Studies have determined that increased social contact can significantly help with depression after a stroke. [20, 21, 23, 24]

Dealing With Exhaustion

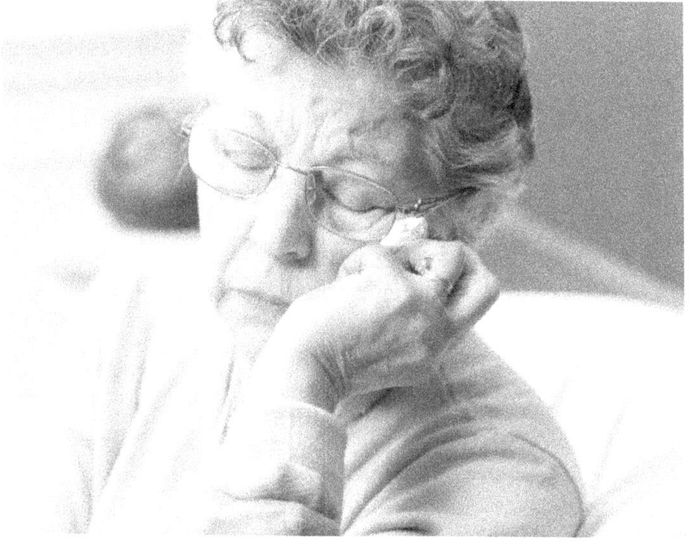

- Movement now requires a lot more energy on your part, when working against resistance, or doing even the simplest repetitions.

- Sweating, panting and an overwhelming urge to stop the activity immediately, are common, even with seemingly easy tasks.

- You may be surprised by how rapidly you become extremely tired.
  You've probably never felt as exhausted as you do when you move the weakened parts of your post-stroke body.

- You'll find that tasks such as getting out of bed, getting in and out of your car and standing for extended periods are a lot harder than they used to be.

- Don't let exhaustion be a disincentive for you to get up and get moving. Frequency is the key.

- Dont get discouraged. Exhaustion is par for the course with stroke rehabilitation. It will get easier. Your stamina will return. The more you do, the stronger you'll become. It's good to recharge with naps.

- You obviously have a lot less stamina than you had pre-stroke, so plan the events in your day according to how much energy you need to expend.

- See your energy as a kind of valuable currency. Once you have spent it, it's gone.

- Conserve your energy. Then when some activity arises unexpectedly, you'll be fine.

- You will learn to siphon out your energy supply with practice. If you have a lunch date, take it easy in the morning. If you exhaust yourself by mid-morning, you'll not feel like going shopping later. After a while you'll get a handle on what you can easily accomplish.

Perfecting Your Gait

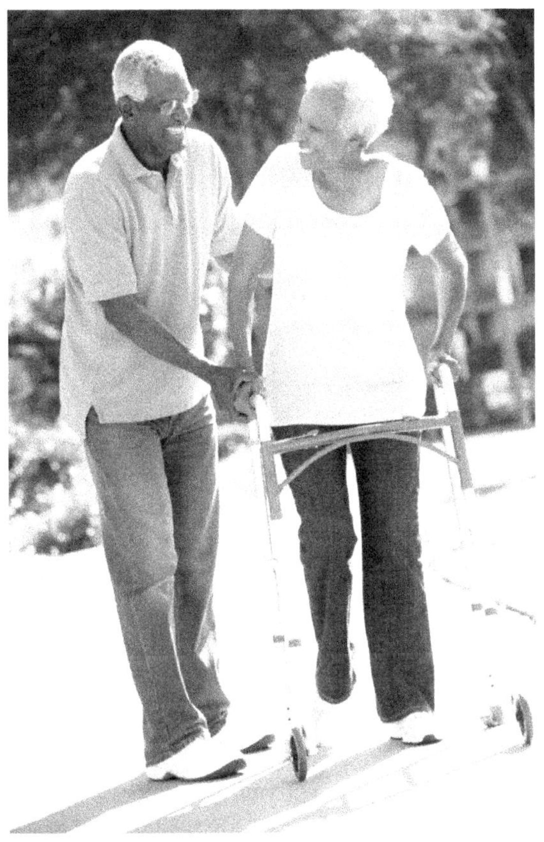

- By working on perfecting your gait, you are retraining your brain, improving your coordination, improving your mobility and reducing the risk of tripping.

- You should focus directly on strengthening the leg on your weak side, lifting your knee, and developing a smooth and rhythmic walking style.

- It's best to take a couple of short walks each day than one long one. You'll actually make better progress.

- Lopsided jerky walking will actually increase your fall risk. Learning to walk with a smooth gait will help your leg regain function quickly.

- When walking with a walker, rollator or cane, focus on lifting the toe of your weak foot when you walk.

- Try to avoid walking flat-footed. Land on your heel, and smoothly bend your foot to your toe before you lift it again for the next step.

- You can do a lot of toe lifts even when you're not walking. Repetitively lift your toe up and down when you're in the car, or while watching television.

- Doing toe-raising exercises at a counter or sink will help strengthen the muscles that lift your foot.. Hang on, lean back on your heels and raise your toes. Do 10 reps twice a day.

- As well as working on strengthening your legs, you should focus directly on improving your balance. So, while grasping a sturdy support, practice putting your weight on your weak leg for 10 seconds at a time.

- Since walking uses a combination of many different muscle groups including your feet, arms, legs, and also your core, add

- The position of your arm is also critical in developing a smooth gait. After the trauma of a stroke, your weak arm is going to automatically curl into your chest in order to "protect" your body.

- Notice the position of your weak arm. Put it down at your side. Straighten out your elbow. You can override the automatic protective arm response by straightening your arm every time you become aware that your elbow is bent.

-

- If you let your arm curl in to your chest, you'll tend to hobble around in a lopsided "stroke walk."

- Realize that arm swings are an integral component of a normal gait. So make a point of swinging your arms.

- Check that your stride for both legs is even, and match your arm swing to the movement of the leg on the opposite side. You'll find that your gait becomes rhythmic and smooth.

- As you walk, swing your weak arm back and imagine an invisible cord linking your weak hand to your weak knee and pulling it up high. Your toe will raise with your knee, and this will help with foot drop.

- Focus on walking smoothly and rhythmically even in your house. Don't allow yourself to slip back into the lop-sided "stroke walk."

- Take it slow and make sure the motion of your walk is smooth. Once you are comfortable with the new process of walking, and feel stable, you'll become less dependent on a cane.

Healing A Subluxed Shoulder

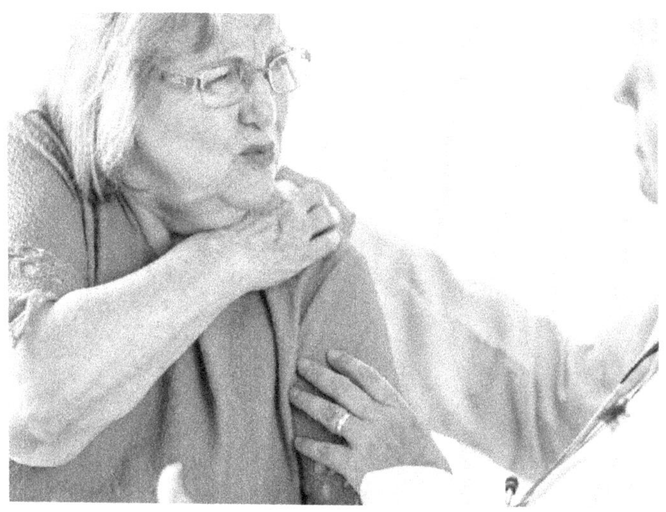

- Be very careful if your shoulder is subluxed and you use a sling, that your hand and shoulder get a daily workout.

- Keeping your shoulder, elbow and hand immobile for days on end is risky because muscle atrophy in your arm and hand can occur quickly when you curtail movement and contracture can result.

- If your shoulder is subluxed, it may help to use kinesthetic tape to support that shoulder. It's important to get the ball of the humerus back up into the shoulder joint.

- At intervals, support your weak arm at the elbow, with your strong arm. Also, support your weak arm by leaning your elbow on the arm rest of your armchair or while riding in your car.

- Move your affected shoulder, arm and wrist only to the point of minor pain. If you go past the pain threshold, it can injure you.

- You can also help subluxation by focusing on using your shoulder muscles to pull your shoulder back in. The best exercise for this is to pull your shoulder blades together as if you are holding a ball between them. Do 20 repetitions per day and your subluxation will diminish.

- Range of motion can be helped by lifting your good arm with your weak arm. Using a pulley, a rod or a cane to lift your weak arm with your strong arm can increase the range of motion in your shoulder. Just remember to stop when it hurts.

Help With Speech Impairment

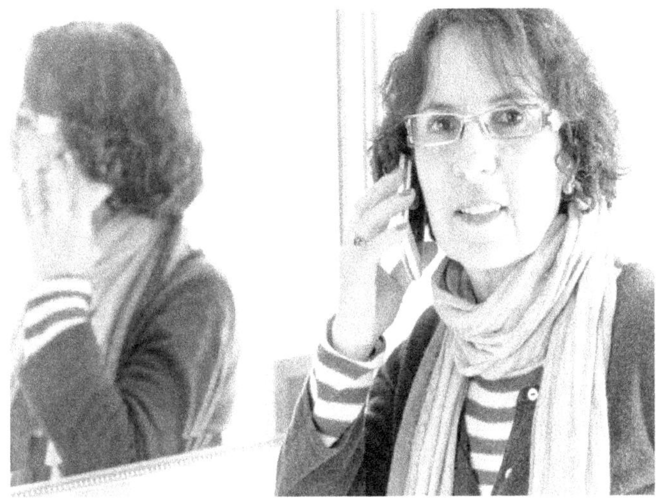

- One common effect of a stroke is aphasia which is an inability to comprehend and express language because of damage to specific areas of the left brain.

- The most common effect of aphasia is taking time to find words. Some people actually lose the ability to speak, comprehend written material, or even write.

- Aphasia is pretty much limited to language difficulties. Intelligence is not affected.

- If you are experiencing difficulty, your doctor can refer you to a speech therapist who has sophisticated techniques for helping you to regain normal speech and help you understand the spoken word more effectively.

- If your speech is affected, focus on speaking as accurately as you can. You may want to employ your tablet or smart phone and use a voice-recognition app to create a journal, to practice speaking accurately, or to make notes of your progress.

- A voice-recognition system such as Dragon Naturally Speaking or Dragon Dictate will actually improve the accuracy of your speech.

- When you pronounce a word incorrectly, a voice recognition system will write the word exactly the way you said it. It is very valuable feedback, and you can simply practice the word until you get it right.

- Repeated studies have established that increased social contact is helpful in reducing aphasia. [17]

- Using language for communication and social interaction significantly reduces chronic aphasia and has been found to be much more effective than practicing speech for long periods (up to 30 hours per week) in a laboratory setting.[17]

Why Nutrition Is Important

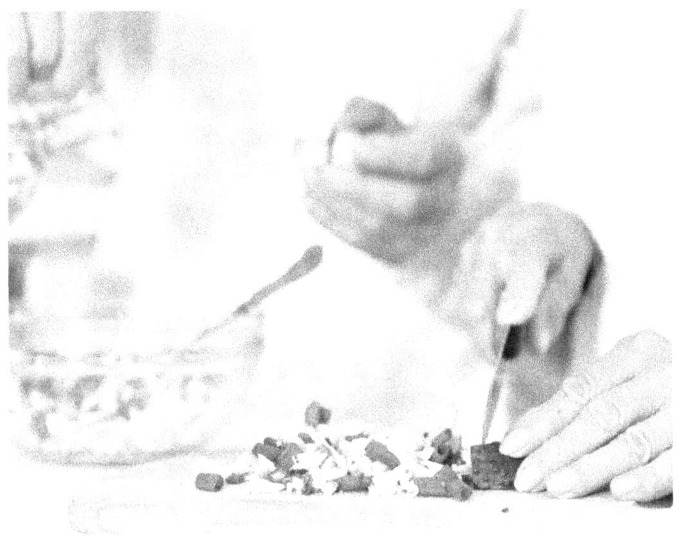

- Enhanced nutrition can really help you. Be aware that as a stroke survivor, you are actually at higher risk for having a second stroke.

- To reduce the risk of another stroke, make sure you follow a healthy diet as recommended by nutritionists, with a minimum of foods containing saturated fat and plenty of colorful veggies.

- Nutrition is important for stroke patients because it is a factor in reducing high blood pressure.

- Lowering your salt intake, remaining hydrated, increasing your potassium intake (eating beans, bananas, acorn squash, avocado, sun dried tomatoes, Swiss chard, dark chocolate and potatoes) can help in normalizing high blood pressure.

- Your body is in the process of healing damaged nerve pathways, atrophied muscles, and infarcted brain tissue. That's quite a project. You will undoubtedly want to get as many phytochemicals into your body as possible.

- Make sure you're eating plenty of colorful and fresh veggies, adequate protein and whole grains.

- There are some nutritional deficiencies that are common in stroke patients. It has been found that serum vitamin D level decreases over time in stroke patients, so vitamin D supplements should be considered.

- One recent study showed that stroke patients who supplemented their diet with vitamin D had statistically less falls. [10]

- Since the brain is composed of nerve cells, your brain, if dried and analyzed, would show a composition of about 30% lecithin.[9]. Lecithin helps the body digest and utilize the fats and oils that are critical in maintaining efficient brain and nerve function which is important after a stroke.

- Nutritionists suggest that the diet of stroke patients be supplemented with lecithin in the form of liquid, capsules, granules or powder added to smoothies and protein shakes. Lecithin is also found naturally in eggs, soy and sunflower seeds.

- Your doctor may refer you to a nutritionist to discuss your eating habits and make sure your diet is not causing any dizziness.

- You are building muscle, so make sure you have enough protein. Protein supplementation in the form of highly efficient protein powders can really boost your daily intake. You might try mixing protein powder with water rather than milk. Since you may have overdone the cholesterol (hello! you had a stroke!)

- You'll probably want to avoid saturated fats, so ease up on the bacon and steak and try a little salmon. If your A1c is high, try to avoid sugar, starches, juices and high glycemic sweeteners.

- Veggies are loaded with minerals which will help the healing process and help you to stay calm.

- Nutritional deficiencies are suspected in stroke patients who experience sudden involuntary jerky movements especially in the legs. These movements, similar to a startle response, are called myoclonus.

- Myoclonic jerks are caused by sudden strong contractions in the muscles of the affected limb. They tend to occur when one is resting or falling asleep. Minor instances are called hypnic jerks.

- Although it is assumed that neural damage is implicated in myoclonus, there is strong evidence that blood calcium levels drop precipitously before myoclonic episodes. [39]

- If you are experiencing frequent myoclonic jerks you may want to consider taking a calcium supplement together with vitamin D to help absorb the calcium. You should check with your doctor to see if taking a calcium supplement would conflict with any of your medications.

- Some researchers take the view that involuntary jerky limb movements are actually the result of B vitamin deficiencies. The medullary sheath surrounding the nerves is composed of lecithin which is a made from choline and inositol, two of the B vitamins.

- Research indicates that B vitamin deficiencies can cause an actual erosion of the medullary sheath which surrounds the nerves, producing little holes in the sheath and enabling electrical impulses to escape into the muscles, causing involuntary contractions. [38]

- Studies have shown that supplementation with vitamin B12 has been found to be very helpful in relieving myoclonus symptoms. [38]

- All stroke survivors should avoid foods that are loaded with cholesterol since high cholesterol could have been a contributing factor to your stroke.

- Also try to avoid refined sugars especially if you're diabetic.

Modifying Your Home

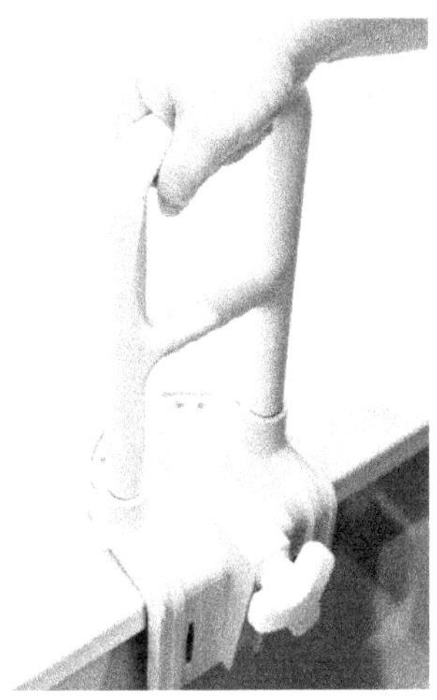

- It is important to adjust your home environment to meet your new needs and reduce the possibility of accidents.

- You may want to have an occupational therapist inspect your home to make sure It Is free of obstructions and safcty hazards and is adequately lit.

- Go around your house and see where you can make improvements. You'll be more able to function in an environment that caters to your needs.

- Keep all doorways and hallways clear and accessible. Place devices that you use for physical therapy in easily accessible locations.

- Remove area rugs and power cords in the living room and kitchen.

- Realize that your bathroom is one of the most common places for falls in the home. Hazards such as slippery wet floors and lightweight rugs increase the risk of falling.

- Transform your bathroom. Use slip-resistant mats in the shower or tub, put in a shower chair, and use a long-handled scrub brush. Replace the shower head with a flexible hose so you can comfortably sit while showering.

- Ask your occupational therapist to check out your bathroom. A well-placed grab bar over the bath can make a big difference.

- Have specific places for your mail, bills, medical receipts, credit cards, cell phone, keys and other items that can be easily misplaced.

- You can keep your home environment tidier and more organized by clearing clutter from counters, having a specific place where everything goes, putting things away directly after use, keeping dishes washed and focusing on keeping up.

- Downsize if necessary. Sell items you no longer need at a garage sale, craigslist, or eBay.

- If you leave items on the floor, you're creating a trip risk. Don't become frustrated, just avoid the risk in the first place by putting items away.

- Make sure charging cable and electrical cables are out of the way so that you don't trip on them.

- The availability of rechargeable very lightweight vacuums makes it easy to keep floors and shelves dust-free, and these can easily be used from a wheel chair.

- You should also make your kitchen more user-friendly. One-handed cutting boards are available, and you can purchase special knives which use vertical force to chop a variety of foods.

- Make sure there are enough chairs readily available so if you suddenly feel the need to sit, a chair or stool is right there.

- If you don't have a dishwasher, use a stool at the sink to wash dishes, and use one at the stove if you find it necessary to cook.

- If you have incontinence or urgency problems you should discuss treatment with your doctor or urologist. Also, if you find that you often need to use the restroom in the middle of the night, make sure the way to the bathroom is lighted, or that you use a bedside commode or urinal.

Be Aware of Possible Drug Interactions

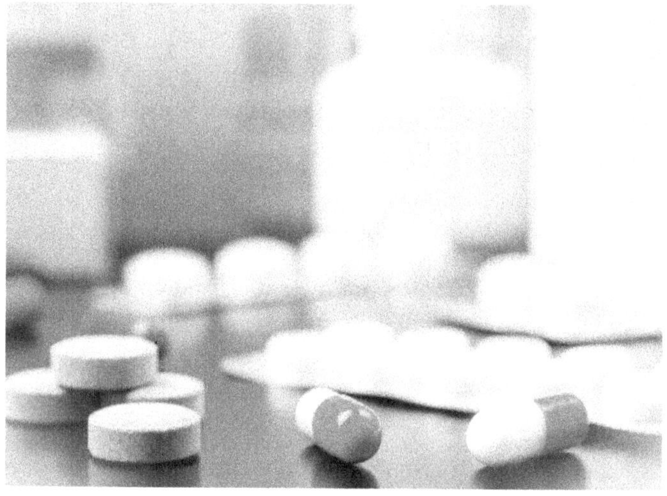

- Make sure that you, your doctor and your caregiver are aware of all the medications you are taking and what each medication does.

- If your blood pressure increases or isn't well-controlled, ask your doctor about alternatives to the medications you are taking. He or she may recommend lifestyle changes as well.

- Also let your doctor know about any vitamin supplements you are taking because some medications and supplements interfere with each other.

- Depending on the medication you are taking, some interactions can be serious. For example, warfarin (a prescription blood thinner), ginkgo biloba (an herbal

- supplement), vitamin E, and aspirin can each thin the blood. Taking any of these together may increase the potential for internal bleeding or another stroke.

- Consuming 200 to 300 milligrams of caffeine can temporarily cause a spike in your blood pressure, but the role caffeine plays in blood pressure is debatable. It's unclear whether the effect is temporary or long lasting.

- For a stroke survivor, maintaining a healthy blood pressure is very important. But some pain and anti-inflammatory medications can conflict with blood pressure medications by causing you to retain water, creating kidney problems and increasing your blood pressure.

- Examples of anti-inflammatory medications are Indomethacin or Indocin, non-steroidal anti-inflammatory drugs (NSAIDs), including naproxen sodium (Aleve, Anaprox) and ibuprofen (Advil, Motrin IB, others), and Piroxicam (Feldene).

- Talk to your doctor about which pain medication is best for you. If you absolutely need to continue taking a pain medication that has been implicated in raising blood pressure, your doctor may recommend an alternate to the medication you are using.

- Antidepressants may also cause an increase in blood pressure. These medications work by affecting brain chemicals including serotonin, norepinephrine and dopamine which impact your mood.

- If you are taking antidepressants, keep aware of your blood pressure. If your blood pressure increases or isn't well-controlled, ask your doctor about alternatives to your current medications.

- Antidepressants that can raise your blood pressure include Venlafaxine (Effexor XR), monoamine oxidase inhibitors, tricyclic antidepressants, and Fluoxetine (Prozac and Saracen).

- For women, birth control pills and other birth control devices contain hormones that may increase your blood pressure by narrowing smaller blood vessels.

- Virtually all birth control pills, patches and vaginal rings come with warnings that high blood pressure may be a side effect. If you already have high blood pressure, consider using a different form of birth control.

- While nearly all birth control pills can raise your blood pressure, your blood pressure may be less likely to increase if you use a birth control pill or device that contains a lower dose of estrogen.

- Decongestants can make some blood pressure medications less effective. They also narrow your blood vessels, which makes it harder for your blood to flow through them and increases blood pressure.

- Decongestants include Pseudoephedrine (Sudafed) and (Neo-Synephrine).

- Check the label of your cold or allergy medication to see if it contains a decongestant. Ask your doctor or pharmacist about over-the-counter cold products made for people who have high blood pressure.

- Some herbal medicines can interfere with medications or directly impact blood pressure. These include Arnica (Arnica montana), Bitter orange (Citrus aurantium), Ephedra (ma-huang), Ginkgo (Ginkgo biloba), Ginseng (Panax quinquefolius and Panax ginseng), Guarana (Paullinia cupana), Licorice (Glycyrrhiza glabra), Senna (Cassia senna) and St. John's wort (Hypericum perforatum).

- Immunosppressants such as Cyclosporine (Neoral, Sandimmune) and Tacrolimus (Prograf) can also. raise blood pressure.

- Stimulants, such as methylphenidate (Ritalin), can raise your blood pressure by causing your heart to beat faster or irregularly.

- A home care agency can help with set up your medicines so you take the right ones, and make sure you are eating well enough.

Your Caregiver Has Needs Too

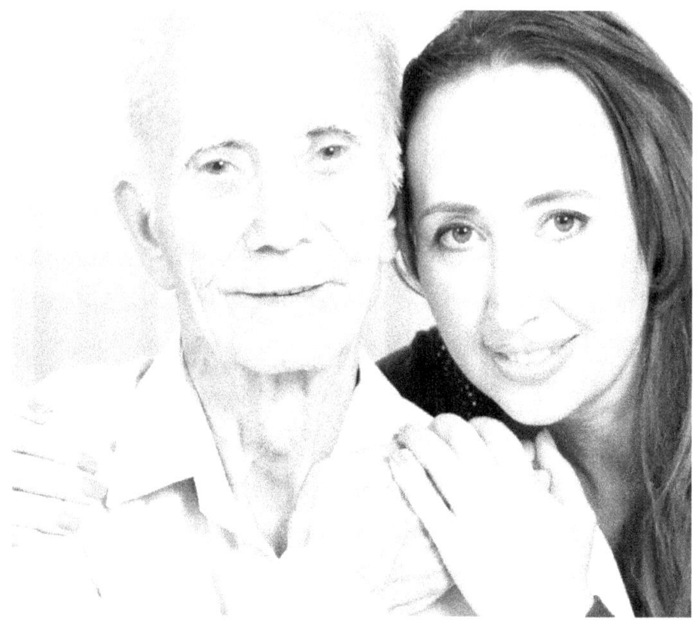

- Be kind to your caregiver. Consider that your caregiver is working on your behalf and be appreciative. The biggest stress for caregivers is that they are not in control of the situation. You are.

- If you're feeling frustrated, angry or depressed, your caregiver can't really do anything other than encourage you and potentially wait it out.

- Encourage your caregiver to take frequent rest breaks and to have social interaction with others. It can be just as stressful to have indirect responsibility and be at the beck and call of a patient, as it is to be the actual patient.

- Make sure that your spouse or caregiver is up to the task of helping you out. If your spouse is not feeling up to par, the task of being your caregiver will seem overwhelming and you may have to opt for hiring someone to help out with meals, dishes and keeping the house tidy.

- Be aware of how stressful being a care-giver can be, especially for a family member. Since not all family relationships are happy ones, stroke patients who have experienced an unhappy past with a caregiver may not realize how stressful it can be for that caregiver, especially if it requires hands-on contact and long hours in your home.

- Old wounds can heal with an attitude of respect, gratitude, cooperation and forgiveness. But it is also possible that those wounds can be inflamed if you are insensitive, unappreciative, demanding or critical.

- Try to create a buddy system with your caregiver. Go for walks together. Do your physical therapy exercises with your caregiver watching and rating you on good form. You'll be more motivated if you are sharing the experience with someone else.

- Consider how much your caregiver is sacrificing and express your appreciation. If you are experiencing friction with your caregiver, it might be time to suggest they take a break and hire a replacement.

- Treat the caregiver as you would a professional rather than the person you've had issues with. You should re-evaluate your relationship with your caregiver in terms of the present, not the past. That was then, this is now. You are getting their help. It's time to appreciate them.

The Importance of Social Contact

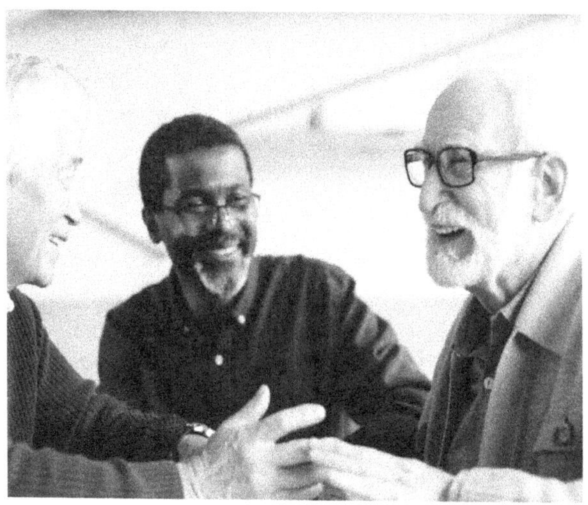

- Studies have found that patients with more social support improve more extensively than those with less support. [17]

- Research indicates that it is patients with milder strokes who are most vulnerable, as friends and family may underestimate their need for social support, leading to a weaker physical recovery. [18]

- Social support not only affects the extent of recovery but also the speed at which it takes place. [18] So make sure you socialize. Don't become isolated.

- You need to go out of your way to be around people. Use your walker. Get a rollator so that you can sit down when you get tired.

- After a month has passed, especially if your left side is affected and right arm and leg are strong, your doctor may be able to give you a letter allowing you to drive. Make it a priority to start driving again. You should try to start driving again, especially if the stroke affected your left side and your right foot is strong.

- Many hospital rehab departments have a computerized system that enables stroke patients to take a simulated driving test and measure reflex times. The machines have a steering wheel, brake and accelerator. It's actually a fun test.

- Once you are driving, get yourself to where people congregate. Maybe, make a point of going to church on Sundays. Go to local concerts. Go to restaurants. Invite friends to share a meal.

- Become attracted to where people are. Go to your local playground and watch the kids play. It's important to feel a part of a group, rather than feeling isolated.

- If you are around other stroke or brain injury victims, encourage them. A smile, a compliment, a word of encouragement will go a long way to making them feel better. And it's likely to ricochet right back to you. A positive force illuminates and heals.

- Prioritize your social needs. Do you need to call a friend to drop by? Do you need to use social media to stay in touch with friends and keep them updated on your progress? Is there more you could be doing to enhance your social network

Managing Stress

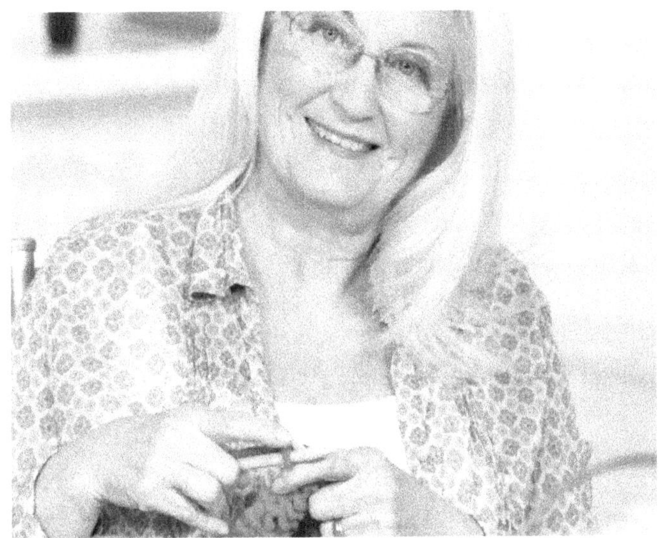

- One important component of stroke recovery is stress reduction. The stress response is a hyper-alert reaction instigated in your body as a reaction to a real or perceived threat.

- Stressors differ from one person to another, but the reaction is remarkably similar. You can tell if you are stressed if you startle easily and are jumpy. Being aware of this is helpful.

- When you are under stress, your body goes into "fight or flight" mode, a lifesaving reaction that has been with humans since caveman days, and it is automatic. No time to think. Just react.

- These days we obviously don't have the threat of dodging wild animals, most of our stress is psychological, but we retain the same archaic stress response of tensing up ready for potential attacks.

- A stress potential for a stroke victim is that your body has already experienced a life-threatening trauma and so you are likely to be subconsciously wary of another threat.

-

- One technique which has been found to be very effective in shutting down the stress response is deep muscle relaxation. This step-by-step process entails progressively "letting go" in all of the muscle groups in your body.

- When combined with very slow deep breathing, deep relaxation has been found to be very effective in training muscles to relax and remain that way.

- Not only does deep relaxation reduce tension, but it also reduces anxiety, the cognitive partner of the stress response. Anxiety is significantly relieved by learning the skill of deep muscle relaxation.

- Learning deep relaxation is easy and can be practiced in 15-minute sessions. Just begin by lying down, then close your eyes and slow your breathing. Count slowly to 5 while breathing in, and slowly to 5 while breathing out. Keep this slow breathing pace during the whole process. Then slowly start relaxing your muscles.

- Visualize your muscles becoming warm, and totally relaxed. Once you're good at relaxing, you'll not only fall asleep after a few minutes, but the residual calming effects will stay with you long after your relaxation session.

- You'll be surprised how easy it is to learn deep relaxation. While slowing your breathing, mentally speak to each muscle group by repeating: "My toes are becoming warm, heavy and relaxed," then "My feet are becoming warm, heavy and relaxed," and so on.

- Start with your toes, then your feet, ankles, calves, and work slowly up your body to your shoulders, neck and scalp. Go up your whole body step-by-step. Also relax the muscles behind your eyes.

- You can't force yourself to relax, you just need to let the relaxation response happen by guiding your body through the process of letting go, and visualizing the muscles becoming warm, heavy and relaxed, one muscle group at a time.

- Practice the deep relaxation protocol at bed time. After you become skilled at deep relaxation, you'll drop off to sleep quickly.

- Clinical studies using an adhesive thermometer attached to the feet of subjects doing deep relaxation and visualizing their feet becoming warmer as they relaxed, showed that this process is quite effective The temperature of the subjects' feet increased several degrees Fahrenheit. [37]

Maintaining A Positive Outlook

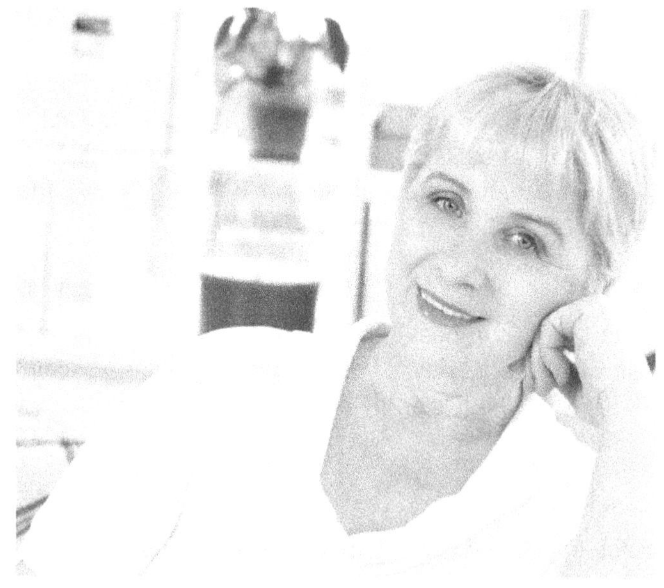

- It's really important that you fully understand just how much influence your mental outlook and attitude have on the speed of your recovery.

- If you take the attitude that your stroke is a challenge that you'll get through, and that you'll emerge stronger and healthier, you probably will.

- If you take the position that life has done you wrong, that you will probably never recover and that this whole mess is totally unfair, you're probably right.

- So figure out where you're at. Success or failure? A blessing or a curse? Negativity or positivity? It's to a large extent up to you.

- Try to catch yourself when you think negatively and see if you can take a positive interpretation of the same thought. For example, " I can't do this," can be reframed as "I'm learning to do this," and "This is too hard," can be turned into "This is hard, but I'm beginning to get it and finding it easier every day."

- When you are worried, use the age-old proven worry formula that highly successful people use. Ask yourself "What is the worst that could happen?" Then face that possible outcome. Accept that this might indeed happen. Now focus on figuring out ways to improve on that outcome.

- Worry is similar to mental chaos. It doesn't improve the situation. It just upsets you and occupies your time. Visualize yourself dealing with solutions to a worry situation. It will give you a roadmap to handling the situation if it happens. You'll find that you will worry less if you focus on solutions.

- You'll find when looking back at your life, that many of the things you worried about the most, didn't actually happen. You wasted a lot of anguish on non-occurrences.

- Do not let your negative thoughts have power over you because those thoughts will end up controlling your life. A mind full of negative thoughts has no room for positivity.

- Remember, negative thoughts crowd out the positive ones. So crowd out every negative thought by looking for the bright side of the situation and do a mental house-cleaning.

- Choose the wrong direction and you can backslide. Choose the right direction and you may be surprised how quickly your body and brain will unite in their effort to get you back to full functionality.

- If you believe that you will fully recover and achieve all the capabilities you had pre-stroke, you undoubtedly will. If you think that life has beaten you down and caused irreparable damage, you'll be right.

- Your recovery speed is to a large extent your choice. Once you make that choice, you will have to accept responsibility for the consequences. Your focus will determine your reality.

- The road to healing will involve some work, some failures, a lot of application and serious discipline.

- Once you achieve normal speech, better memory, full balance, the ability to walk normally and the full use of your affected hand and arm, you will be very grateful for the direction you chose.

- Life is too short to waste your time with situations that don't lift you up and support you and people who don't love and respect you.

- Make sure the mental and emotional climate you surround yourself with is positive and reinforcing. The people you have contact with and even the TV shows you watch are likely to impact you.

- Positive thinking is merely a habit. You have the time now to get it right. The more positive you are, the faster you'll heal your mind and body, and the more socially attractive you will be.

- Sometimes you need to go through a phase of being challenged in order to learn and grow, and the most efficient path may not be the most easy one for you. You may have to step out of your comfort zone to heal.

- Remember, this journey is not just in your mind. Your injured body is like an reluctant child and must be guided accordingly.

- It is during times of adversity that we grow. To really appreciate your good health, you sometimes need to have it forcibly removed for a while.

- The more you have confidence and appreciation of your true self, the less affected you'll be by bumps in the road.

- Ask yourself which is the biggest benefit you've gotten from having had your stroke. Seriously. Only you can figure out the way that your stroke impacted you in a positive way.

- If you can't figure it out, ask yourself again before you go to bed, and sleep on it. There is a benefit, but it's up to you to find out what it is.

- Now that you are dealing with the after-effects of your stroke, you'll probably be more empathetic to other disabled people. You may also realize that your life is potentially richer, more meaningful and clearer than it was before.

Time to Make Some Lifestyle Changes

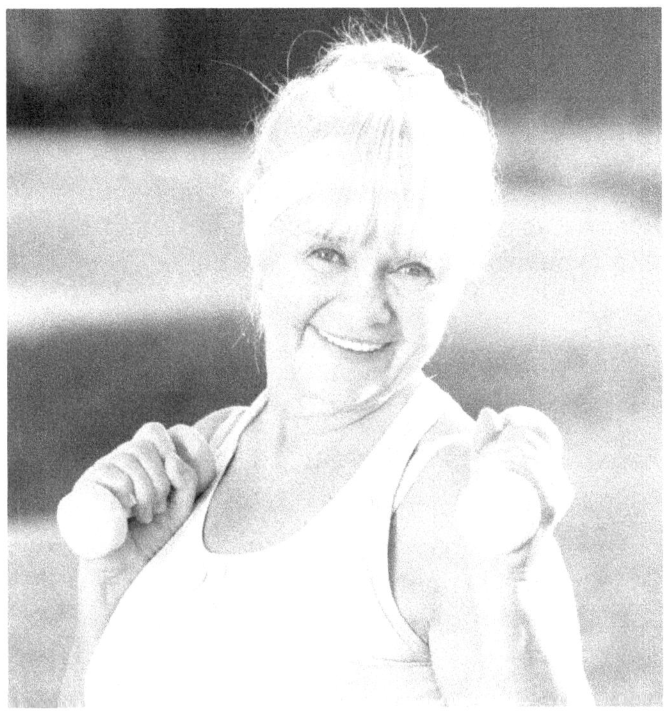

- You woke up after having your stroke as a new person. By surviving your stroke, life has given you a second chance.

- What changes are you going to make? You have been to the precipice and come back. How are you going to make this life-changing experience beneficial to you? What are you going to dispense with and what are you going to add to make your life more fulfilling?

- Examine your beliefs, attitudes and behavior and see if you can figure out a way to worry less, experience less anxiety, replace rigid out-of-date beliefs and embrace positivity and freedom of thought.

- Now's the time to examine grudges and drop them, to become kinder, to empathize with others rather than focusing on you, to treat your body well, to eat better, to exercise daily. Life is more meaningful when you try harder.

- Realize that your lifestyle has changed—not permanently—but for long enough to re-evaluate where you're going with your life.

- Play it cool. It's easy to become frustrated when it takes so much longer to do simple tasks, when you drop things, when getting in and out of a car seems just so much more of an effort than it used to be, but this is the card you've been dealt. Hey, you lived through it.

- Talk to your doctor, your physical therapist, a nutritionist and if you are diabetic, an endocrinologist. Force change on yourself. Don't repeat the same old erroneous patterns of behavior that brought you to this point.

- Move more. If you weren't very active before you had the stroke, try and make the change to a more active lifestyle.

- Eat better. Keep tabs on your cholesterol and A1c levels. Think in positive terms. Erase hate and negativity. Your stroke will become a life-changing event in a good way.

- Having survived a stroke means that you probably had a scare. In anticipation of stent surgery, or balloon angioplasty, you may have thought about the possibility of dying. So how has that impacted your life?

- Have you considered where you're at in terms of the legacy you're creating? Is your stroke an opportunity to make changes?

- Perhaps an event that others could perceive as horrendous, may in fact be your catalyst for adapting to a new reality, a new you.

- Make a list of the things that make you feel uncomfortable. Is it the pain? Is it the fact that you're physically limited? Is it the exhaustion? Is it the social isolation? You are going to have your own unique list. Now focus on solutions.

- Create the best life possible. You deserve it. Keep in mind that you have three things going for you. 1) you have a great reason to rest as much as you want; 2) you have the potential to become completely healed; 3) more medical breakthroughs on stroke rehab are happening every month.

- What do you truly believe in? What is it going to take for you to love yourself? What is important in your life? Who are your true friends?, what do you enjoy doing best? What have you always wanted to do, but put off? You might be surprised at the answers you get when you start asking yourself these important questions.

- You were spared for a reason. Now it's time to live the rest of your life differently. What changes will you have to make to survive physically, mentally and emotionally?

- Your stroke will certainly slow you down, but that may not be a bad thing. Take the time you have now to re-evaluate your life. Can you be more patient? Can you be kinder and more empathetic—especially to other disabled people?

- Take this time to reconsider your life goals. What's important? Money? Career? Accumulating more stuff? The answers will become obvious.

- A life-changing adversity such as a stroke can seriously impact a person, but adversity is a necessary element of individual growth and can actually reveal our true potential.

- We are stronger when we endure and overcome challenges and move forward. Never lose hope. Storms make us stronger and never last forever.

- If you believe you are a victim and that life is unfair, you will be less proactive in fixing the conditions that led to your stroke. You obviously can't change the past, but you can make changes now.

- The Copenhagen City Heart Study of 2,000 stroke survivors over 30 years, revealed that life expectancy after stroke actually increased more than that of the general population.[4]

Why? Because the stroke survivors made some lifestyle changes and extended their life expectancy.

- You might want to take an objective look at the level of stress you were experiencing before your stroke, your pre-stroke cholesterol and A1c numbers, how much exercise you were getting, the percentage of fresh vegetables in your diet and how many hours per day you spent in front of the TV.

- How can you improve your cholesterol or A1c numbers now if you think they might not have been really working for you? Talk to your doctor or caregiver, he or she may come up with some suggestions you never thought of.

New Breakthroughs in Stroke Research

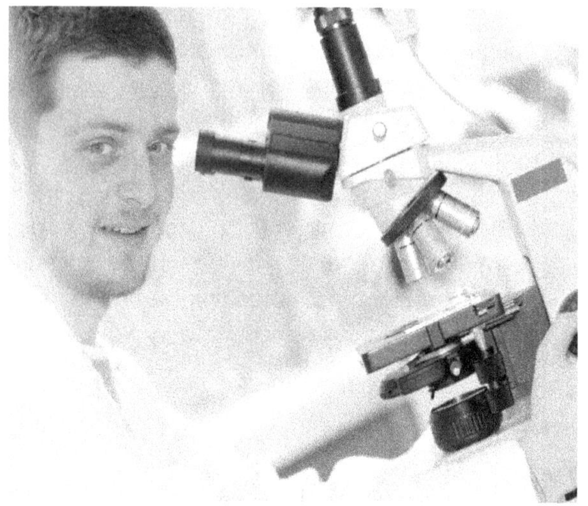

- Stroke rehabilitation has now progressed to a point where improvement is predictable and reliable.

- New techniques in physical therapy related to the function of specific muscles and range of motion, have rapidly increased recovery time, allowing patients to achieve pre-stroke functionality more rapidly than was even imagined in recent decades. [2, 27]

- Because there are so many aging baby boomers, an increasing number of people suffer from strokes every year, and there is more funding for research.

- Stroke is now the second leading cause of death globally. Each year 795,000 Americans have strokes. Of those, 140,000 die, and 185,000 have secondary strokes. [3]

- Because of the massive increase in the number of people having strokes, there has also been a corresponding explosion of medical research focused on stroke recovery.

- The future of stroke rehabilitation remains one of promise and challenge in treating residual disabilities, especially for testing biological interventions for neural repair in the most seriously affected patients. [36]

- Many leading stroke rehabilitation centers are using technological breakthroughs to increase gains in performance at any time after a stroke. [36]

- The Copenhagen City Heart Study of 20,000 men and women followed 2000 first-time stroke survivors over a 30 year period from 1978. During that time, 37% died from another stroke, 28% from heart disease, 12% from cancer and 23% from other causes. For those 65 to 72, 11% survived 15 years, for those under 65, 28% survived 15 years. [6.]

- A most interesting statistic from the Copenhagen Study showed that improved after-stroke care increased life expectancy up to 4 years during the period from 1978 to 2001.[6] This actually exceeded the increase in life expectancy of the general population. [5] Wow!

- This statistic should be super encouraging to stroke survivors who are willing to make lifestyle changes. You've got time to forge ahead into a new life

- When you have a stroke and survive the first month, your likelihood of dying during the first year after the stroke is about 10%. Be aware that as a stroke survivor, your risk of having a second stroke in the next 10 years is 43%, but changes in lifestyle can dramatically improve that probability. [1,5]

- High blood pressure is a leading cause of secondary strokes. But changes in lifestyle and proactive behavior can reduce your risk significantly. [1]

- Stroke recovery is actually measurable on a scale called the Functional Independence Measure Score. This test is the standard for patients in stroke rehabilitation facilities. Patients are expected to improve several points per week.

- Patients are measured on motor capacities including: 1) self-care—eating, grooming, bathing, dressing, toileting; 2) sphincter control— bowel and bladder; 3) transfers — bed, chair, wheelchair, toilet, tub, shower; and 4) locomotion—walking, using a wheelchair and using stairs. [8]

- Stroke patients are also rated on cognitive capacity including 1) communication—comprehension and expression; and 2) social cognition—social interaction, problem solving and memory. Scores are also impacted by whether the patient can accomplish these tasks independently or whether the patient needs a helper.

- If you are recovering from your stroke at home, you may want to keep these criteria in mind when assessing how well you are doing.[8]

- Experimental therapies at leading stroke research centers include non-invasive brain stimulation. Techniques such as transcranial magnetic stimulation have been used with some success in a research setting to help improve a variety of motor skills.[36]

- In some experimental facilities, therapies such as stem cells, are being investigated, but can only be used as part of a clinical trial. [35]

- Alternative medicine techniques are also being researched. Treatments such as massage, herbal therapy, acupuncture and oxygen therapy are being evaluated.[30,31]

- Some of these technological innovations include functional electrical stimulation where electricity is applied to weakened muscles, causing them to contract. The electrical stimulation may help re-educate muscles to normal functionality.

- Robotic devices are also being used by leading stroke centers. Robotic technology can assist impaired limbs perform repetitive motions, helping the limbs to regain strength and function.[28]

- Some stroke centers use wireless activity monitors to encourage patients to increase post-stroke activity. [35]

- Virtual reality is also being used in some state-of-the-art stroke centers. The use of video games and other computer-based therapies enables stroke patients to interact with a simulated, real-time environment.[28]

- If you are living near a large population area, you may have access to technology that may not be an option if you live in a small country town, but even if you live far from a stroke center, the new breakthroughs in physical therapy will help you.

- If you focus on repetitive movement and strengthening your weak areas, using a resistance band, a pulley, light weights, and a squishy ball, you will be able to recover efficiently and fast.

- Even if you do not have access to a stroke center, you can benefit from new research.

- An effective and inexpensive technique for increasing mobility in stroke rehabilitation was recently established by a Taiwanese study at National Chiao Tung University. The researchers used thermal stimulation — alternate applications of heat and cold — and found that this significantly improved the function of paralyzed arms and hands of stroke patients. [7]

- Thermal stimulation works by simultaneously activating large areas of the brain which can be beneficial for functional reorganization and neural plasticity and can be helpful for readjusting motor control circuitry. Thermal stimulation is standard practice in orthopedic rehabilitation, and it is also used to treat dysphagia, difficulty in swallowing, that can be caused by a stroke or other conditions. [7]

- The Taiwanese study was the first reported trial of the method in stroke rehabilitation. The trial included 46 stroke patients. Half got standard rehabilitation therapy, the other half standard treatment plus thermal stimulation. Those patients had five sessions a day for six weeks. Each session lasted 20 to 30 minutes, with alternate applications to a hand and wrist of a cold pack, with a temperature just above freezing, alternated with a hot pack. [7]

- Thermal stimulation was found to have a psychological effect. The enhancement of voluntary movement of the paralyzed hand created hope in the stroke patients and this psychological driving force encouraged recovery.

- The thermal stimulation patients had significantly better numbers on four of six measures of function, including changes in sensation, grasping strength and ability to bend the wrist. The researchers are presently using the technique to treat stroke patients. [7]

- Recent clinical trials provide evidence for a range of new interventions to manage walking, reach and grasp, aphasia, visual field loss, and inattention.[36]

- As more and more studies and experimental trials uncover the most efficient methods for healing, rehabilitation is now very predictable. With the help of applied science in physical and occupational therapy, full recovery is now possible. But research shows that it needs patient participation and it won't happen automatically. [35]

References

1. American Heart Association, American Stroke Association, *About Stroke*, strokeassociation.org, 10/23/2012
2. Dobkin BH, Dorsch A. *New evidence for therapies in stroke rehabilitation*. Current atherosclerosis reports. 2013;15(6):331. doi:10.1007/s11883-013-0331y.
3. Law M, Wald N, Morris J. *Lowering blood pressure to prevent myocardial infarction and stroke: a new preventive strategy*. 2003. In: NIHR Health Technology Assessment programme: Executive Summaries. Southampton (UK): NIHR Journals Library.
4. Mukhtar, O., & Jackson, S. H. D. (2013). *Risk: benefit of treating high blood pressure in older adults*. British Journal of Clinical Pharmacology, 2018, 75(1), 36–44..
5. U.S. centers for Disease Control and Prevention, published by The Internet Stroke Center.
6. Aguib Y, Al Suwaidi J. *The Copenhagen City Heart Study (Østerbroundersøgelsen)*. Global Cardiology Science & Practice. 2015;2015(3):33. doi:10.5339/gcsp.2015.33.
7. Jia-Ching Chon, Chung-Chao Liang and Fu-Zen Shaw, *Facilitation of Sensory and Motor Recovery by Thermal Intervention for the Hemiplegic Upper Limb in Acute Stroke Patients: A Single-Blind Randomized Clinical Trial,* Stroke. 2005;36:2665-2669; November 3, 2005;
8. *Functional Independence Measure* (FIM) The FIM was developed in 1983 by a task force created by the American Congress of Rehabilitation Medicine and the American Academy of Physical Medicine and Rehabilitation headed by Carl Granger and Byron Hamilton [11].Nov 29, 2009
9. Dianne Craft, MA, CNHP, *Improving Your Memory With Lecithin, Nov 2, 2017*
10. Shuba Narasimhan and Prakash Balasubramanian, *Role of Vitamin D in the Outcome of Ischemic Stroke- A Randomized Controlled Trial,* Journal of Clinical and Diagnostic Research, 2017.

11. Lim JY, Jung SH, Kim WS, Paik NJ. *Incidence and risk factors of post stroke falls after discharge from inpatient rehabilitation.*PM R. 2012 Dec; 4(12):945-53. Epub 2012 Sep 6.

12. Laura M Wagner, Victoria L Phillips, [...], and Pamela G Forducey. *Falls among community-residing stroke survivors following inpatient rehabilitation: a descriptive analysis of longitudinal data.* BMC Geriatrics. 2009;9:46. doi:10.1186/1471-2318-9-46.

13. Tsur A1, Segal Z., *Falls in stroke patients: risk factors and risk management.* Isr Med Assn Journal. 2010 Apr;12(4):216-9.

14. Marlies R. de Jong, Maarten Van der Elst, and Klaas A. Hartholt, *Drug-related falls in older patients: implicated drugs, consequences, and possible prevention strategies,* Departement of Surgery, Reinier de Graafweg 3-11, 2625 AD Delft, The Netherlands; Ther Adv Drug Saf. 2013 Aug; 4(4): 147–154.

15. Elles Douven, Sebastian Köhler, [...], and Pauline Aalten, *Imaging Markers of Post-Stroke Depression and Apathy: a Systematic Review and Meta-Analysis,* Neuropsychol Rev. 2017; 27(3): 202–219.

16. Amy Quilty OT Reg. (Ont.), Occupational Therapist, *Cognitive Behaviour Therapy (CBT) and Stroke Rehabilitation,* Cognitive Behavioural Therapy (CBT) Certificate Program, University of Toronto, Quinte Health Care.

17. Jonathon Prousky, *Niacinamide's Potent role in Alleviating Anxiety with its Benzodiazepine-like Properties*: A Case Report. Orthomolecular Health. 10/28/2008.

18. Shahmansouri N, Farokhnia M, Abbasi SH, et al S. *A randomized, double-blind, clinical trial comparing the efficacy and safety of Crocus sativus L. with fluoxetine for improving mild to moderate depression in post percutaneous coronary intervention patients.* J Affect Disord. 2013 Nov 16. doi:pii: S0165-0327(13)00797-0.

19. Brian D. Lawenda, M.D., *Saffron Extract Works As Well As Prozac For Depression,* Mar 2, 2015

20. Glass, T.A., Matchar, D.B., Belyea, M. & Feussner, J.R. (1993). *Impact of social support on outcome in first stroke.* Stroke, 24, 64–70.

21. Saltera, K., Foleya, N. & Teasella, R. (2010). *Social support interventions and mood status post stroke: A review.* International Journal of Nursing Studies, 47(5), 616–625.

22. Åström, M., Adolfsson, R. & Asplund, K. (1993). *Major depression in stroke patients: A 3-year longitudinal study.* Stroke, 24, 976–982.

23. Morris, P., Robinson, R., Raphael, B. & Bishop, D. (1991). *The relationship between the perception of social support and post-stroke depression in hospitalized patients.* Psychiatry, 54, 306–316.

24. Tsouna-Hadjis, E., Vemmos, K., Zakopoulos, N. & Stamatelopoulos, S. (2000*). First-stroke recovery process: The role of family social support.* Archives of Physical Medicine and Rehabilitation, 81(7), 881–887.

25. *"Behavior Changes After Stroke,"* appearing in the Stroke Connection Magazine January/February 2005. (Last science update March 2013) Daroff RB, et al. Neurological rehabilitation. In: Bradley's Neurology in Clinical Practice. 7th ed. Philadelphia, Pa.: Saunders Elsevier; 2016. https://www.clinicalkey.com. Accessed March 28, 2017.

26. Bope ET, et al. *The nervous system.* In: Conn's Current Therapy 2017. Philadelphia, Pa. Elsevier; 2017. https://www.clinicalkey.com. Accessed March 28, 2017.

27. AskMayoExpert. *Stroke rehabilitation.* Rochester, Minn.: Mayo Foundation for Medical Education and Research; 2017.

28. Fu MJ, et al. *Stroke rehabilitation using virtual environments.* Physical Medicine & Rehabilitation Clinics of North America. 2015;26:747.

29. Cunningham DA, et al. *Tailoring brain stimulation to the nature of rehabilitative therapies in stroke.* Physical Medicine & Rehabilitation Clinics of North America. 2015;26:759.

30. *Stroke.* Natural Medicines Accessed April 24, 2017 http://naturalmedicines.therapeuticresearch.com.

31. *Oxygen therapy*. Natural Medicines. Accessed April 24, 2017. http://naturalmedicines.therapeuticresearch.com.
32. *Stroke rehabilitation information*. National Institute of Neurological Disorders and Stroke. https://www.ninds.nih.gov/Disorders/All-Disorders/NINDS-Stroke-Information-Page/Stroke-Rehabilitation-Information. Accessed March 28, 2017.
33. Hoenig H. *Program components and settings for rehabilitation*. http://www.uptodate.com/home. March 28, 2017.
40. Hoenig H. *Patient assessment and common indications for rehabilitation*. http://www.uptodate.com/home. March 28, 2017.
41. Schultz BA (expert opinion). Mayo Clinic, Rochester, Minn. April 23, 2017.
42. Mayo Clinic Staff. Stroke rehabilitation: *What to expect as you recover*. May 24,2017
43. Kristin Lund, *Warm feet relaxation method improves blood flow to the feet*, July 20, 2009
44. de Souza A, Moloi MW. *Involuntary movements due to vitamin B12 deficiency*. Neurol Res. 2014 Dec; 36(12):1121-8.
45. R. Thiel, Ph.D., *Might Calcium Disorders Cause or Contribute to Myoclonic Seizures?* Med Hypotheses; 2006; 66(5):969-74.Epub 2006 Jan 24.
46. Jodi Edwards, Ph.D., affiliate investigator, Ottawa Hospital Research Institute, and Sunnybrook Health Sciences Center, Toronto, Ontario, Canada; Anand Patel, M.B.B.S., vascular neurologist, Northwell Health Neuroscience Institute, Manhasset, N.Y.; Michael Hill, M.D., professor, neurology, University of Calgary, Canada; *Stroke survivors risk* July 24, 2017, Canadian Medical Association Journal
47. Vital Signs: *Recent trends in stroke death rates – United States, 2000-2015*. MMWR 2017; 66.
48. Benjamin EJ, Blaha MJ, Chiuve SE, et al. on behalf of the American Heart Association Statistics Committee and Stroke Statistics Subcommittee. *Heart disease and stroke statistics—2017* update: a report from the American Heart Association. Circulation. 2017;135:e229-e445.

49. Hall MJ, Levant S, DeFrances CJ. *Hospitalization for stroke in U.S. hospitals, 1989–2009*. NCHS data brief, No. 95. Hyattsville, MD: National Center for Health Statistics; 2012.

50. Fang J, Keenan NL, Ayala C, Dai S, Merritt R, Denny CH. *Awareness of stroke warning symptoms—13 states and the District of Columbia*, 2005. MMWR 2008;57:481–5.

51. Executive Summary: Heart Disease and Stroke Statistics—2016 Update

52. Dariush Mozafarian, et al, *Dietary guidelines and health—is nutrition science up to the task? BMJ* 2018;360:k822, Mar 16, 2018;

53. Eric L. Ding, Dariush Mozafarian,*Optimal dietary habits for the prevention of stroke*, Seminars in Neurology, 26 (1) 11-23 March 2006.

54. Hopkinsmedicine.org, *Three Ways to Avoid a Second Stroke*, June 2, 2018